INTRODUCTION AND ORIENTATION
TO
<u>INTEGRATED MEDICINE</u>

SECOND EDITION

Dr. Amol V. Javdekar

M.B.B.S , M.D (Pathology)

DEDICATED TO

All doctors in service of mankind

PREFACE TO SECOND EDITION

While working as a medical officer in ESIS dispensary way back in 1997 I happened to meet a few patients who reported astonishing clinical benefits after taking ***Ayurvedic and homeopathic treatments***. This kindled my interest in trying to know more about these 2 pathies – which are traditionally referred to as ***"alternative medicine"***, ***Allopathy or modern medicine*** being referred to as ***"conventional medicine "***. My scientific study of Homeopathy began in 1998 and of Ayurveda in 2015 and has been ongoing ever since.

I was fortunate to have been primarily trained as a modern medicine doctor (M.B.B.S and M.D in Pathology) from B.J. Medical College , Pune and thus have sound knowledge of basic sciences , especially physiology , pathology , microbiology and modern pharmacology This knowledge and practical experience as a pathologist helped me immensely to scientifically evaluate the response to treatment ever since I started treating patients some time in 2016 using a judicious combination of Allopathy , Ayurveda and Homeopathy.

As my experience grew I started understanding the finer nuances of use of each pathy - the pros and cons / advantages and disadvantages / efficacies and limitations of all 3 pathies. Honest feedback from patients – both positive and negative - about my treatment helped me separate hard facts from tall claims.

By 2021 , after having studied Allopathy for about 29 years , Homeopathy for about 23 years and Ayurveda for about 6 years , I decided to share my knowledge in the form of this book with medical fraternity . This book contains accumulated wisdom borne out of careful application of principles of each of the 3 pathies to real life patients. Even then I do not expect each and every doctor to agree with each and every statement I have made in this book. Differences of opinion are bound to be there considering the extremely high complexity of medicine as a science , its intricacies and subjectivities.

The aim of this book is to introduce and orient the readers to integrated medicine – the necessity of which has been felt by many doctors over past numerous years. Aim is certainly not to teach medicine to anyone since that would need a separate much bigger book. If , after reading this book , **practising doctors get a new insight into potential of integrated medicine in improving patient care , patients understand the options available in front of them and government authorities take urgent steps to start well funded research into this field** I believe the book would have served its purpose.

I have tried to keep the language as simple as possible so that even non medicos can benefit from this book. If a myth is oft repeated for a long time people tend to accept it as a truth. This book will dispel important myths widely prevalent in general public about all 3 pathies.

At the end of this book , in the bonus section , readers will find 6 articles I have written on various aspect of pathology testing , doctor patient relationship and interaction of patients with healthcare in general. Hope readers benefit a lot from these as well.

I am extremely indebted to many homeopaths who helped me understand its intricacies. Special thanks to **Dr. Ajit Kulkarni** (internationally famous homeopath stalwart with 40 books to his credit and recipient of "Homeo Ratna") , **Dr. K. C. Shah** (senior teacher of Homeopathy with 40 years of teaching experience) and **Dr. Pushkar Godbole** who happens to be a brilliant student of Dr. K.C. Shah.

From the Ayurvedic side , special thanks to **Dr. Poonam Phal** , **Dr. Jyoti Mundargi** , **Dr. Prayag Sethiya** for providing much needed guidance regarding usage of Ayurvedic medicines **and Dr. Chandrakumar Deshmukh** for showing ayurvedic parasurgical techniques.

Special thanks to publishing team of Notion Press for their guidance and co – operation during international publishing of this book

- ### *What is new in second edition ?*

(1) Extensive revision of chapter on Ayurveda with information about how Ayurveda can be effectively used even in emergency situations.
(2) Addition of 2 new things to chapter on homeopathy : Word on Biochemic remedies and word on Bach flower remedies.
(3) Guidance of which pathy to use in which disease.

Happy reading !!

-- **Dr. Amol Javdekar**
M.D (Pathology)

FOREWORD FROM DR. AJIT KULKARNI

Dr Amol Javdekar's treatise on " Introduction and Orientation to Integrated Medicine" is a welcome addition to the healers of Medicine who want to treat their patients in a holistic way.

Dr Amol Javdekar, M.D. (Pathology) is a well-known figure not only in Pune but also in India. He is famous for his teachings of various subjects of medicine amongst the students and practitioners of all the three major systems of Medicine viz. Allopathy, Ayurveda and Homeopathy through thoroughly prepared charts, slides and CDs.

Dr Amol is acquainted with me since the last 23 years and I remember when we met first when he was a student of MBBS. He came to meet me at Satara from Pune to discuss some of his queries about Homeopathy. My first impression about this dynamic and inquisitive student was that Dr Amol would find his way in his life and he would create a niche for himself. In the true sense, he is in an ever-expanding state of openness and diligence. He is a knowledge-hunter and his appetite for realization of healing approaches with their variable philosophical bases have not limited him to engage himself only to the mainstream medicine.

The walls of "call me great 24/7" , "dogmatism" , and "we are the only scientific community on the planet" don't imprison the dynamic personality of Dr. Amol. Change is the only constant variable in life and Medicine must accept the variations, vagaries and modifications which occur in the process of evolution for the sake of catering to the needs of suffering of the human beings. No conscientious physician can remain neutral to the developments occurring in all medical faculties.

Truth searching physicians like Dr Amol Javdekar try to look at the field of Medicine through a wide lens of integrated medicine. Dr Amol understands that the time has come to integrate all the faculties to allay sufferings of mankind.

Certain inferences given by the author under the chapter "Homeopathy" are noteworthy :

- Homeopathy has shown to benefit unconscious, semi-conscious patients, infants, animals like dogs, cats and even plants. In all these categories of subjects, placebo effect is just not relevant. Disappearance of visible structural problems like warts, healing of ulcers which previously were not healing are sure shot evidences that Homeopathy acts beyond placebo effect.
- The sceptics of Homeopathy say that there is no research in Homeopathy. They probably do so because of lack of knowledge of research studies being done to elucidate mechanisms of Homeopathy.

- Homeopathy is a gentle and effective form of treatment which stimulates the natural ability of the organism to heal itself.
- Since Homeopathy uses "simple substances in micro-doses, medicines are not associated with any toxicological effect and can be safely used for pregnant women and lactating mothers, infants and children and in the geriatric population.

Many such gems can be quoted from this important book and the author has presented an honest unbiased view of the whole theme of integration with merits and demerits , pros and cons.

The integrated approach to the indivisible individual in terms of patient care management and medical education is the need of the hour. Dr Amol renders a strong message to the physicians of all pathies to be open minded and oriented, to be unbiased and unprejudiced, to be integrated and enlightened; for, every physician's ultimate aim is to mitigate the suffering to preserve and restore the health.

Dr Amol must be complimented for his contemplative analysis of the three pathies with their scope and limitations and for his humane approach to the subject of integration in Medicine at such a time when the world is engulfed by the variants of viruses when unpredictability matters the most for the human species.

DR. AJIT KULKARNI M.D. (HOM.)

- Director, Homeopathic Research Institute, Pune
- A veteran homoeopath, an academician and a famed international teacher
- Co-Author: Absolute Homoeopathic Matera Medica
- Five Regional Repertories: AIDS, DM, Thyroid, HTN and Trauma
- Author:
    - Law of Similars in Medical Science
    - Homeopathic Posology
    - Kali Family and Its Relations
    - Body Language and Homeopathy
    - Homeopathy through Harmony and Totality Three volumes
    - Homeopathic Covidoscope (published by Amazon)
- Has given around 100 international seminars in different parts of the world
- Awards : 'Excellence in Homoeopathy' , 'Homeo-Ratna' , 'Life achievement Award' , 'Dr. B. Sahni Memorial Award'
- Member of editorial board of National Journal Of Homeopathy , Mumbai.

FOREWORD FROM DR. K. C. SHAH

Since my wife , who herself is a pathologist , used to refer samples to the diagnostic centre where Dr. Amol Javdekar works as a pathologist , he was known to me as a pathologist who gave excellent quality path reports. So it came as a surprise for me when one day he visited me to get his doubts regarding Homeopathy clarified. He had systematically categorized his doubts and from the level of his queries it was obvious to me that I was not dealing with a novice in Homeopathy but an allopath who had phenomenal depth of understanding of complexities of Homeopathy. In fact , even after all my 40 years of experience in teaching Homeopathy I admit that I could not clarify few of his doubts and in fact got an insight into certain aspects of Homeopathy.

While discussing various complexities pertaining to some of his patients , Dr. Amol would readily accept most of my suggestions and politely discuss others where he felt otherwise. What I liked was he would always phone his patients to carefully monitor response to treatment and give me feedback wherever necessary. Needless to say , confidentiality of the patient was totally maintained in all these discussions.

Pathology itself is a very vast subject. Attempting to be a clinician together with a pathologist is a daunting task. And being a pathologist and having satisfactorily deep knowledge of Allopathy , Ayurveda and Homeopathy is unbelievable and unheard of. I know of Ayurvedic and Homeopathic doctors who routinely practice Allopathy (in addition to their own pathy) and few allopaths who practice Homeopathy. But a pathologist involved in lab work and handling such wide range of patients is …… as I said ….. unheard of.

So when Dr. Amol told me that he was going to write a book on Integrated Medicine I felt it was very apt and quite within his scope of expertise. I have gone through excerpts of this book and feel it has been very nicely written. Certain analogies he has given to explain certain practices in Homeopathy are not mentioned anywhere else and are his contribution to field of Homeopathy.

Considering the trend these days of patients trying to seek treatment from doctors of all pathies it has become important for doctors from all pathies to have atleast a basic orientation to the opportunities and challenges that this trend poses in clinical practice.

I hope all doctors welcome this book with an open mind , non medicos also benefit from information written in this book and government authorities take steps to fund research in integrated medicine. Best luck to Dr. Amol for any future endeavours.

DR. K. C. Shah L.C.E.H , B.H.M.S , M.D (Hom)

FOREWORD FROM DR. POONAM PHAL

I have known Dr. Amol Javdekar for about 18 months only and what impressed me was his earnestness to conduct in depth study on his own on Ayurveda and Homeopathy in addition to Allopathy (of which he has a formal degree) and to put it in print to give his readers an entirely new dimension regarding integration of these 3 pathics.

From the numerous discussions we have had over telephone regarding various aspects of Ayurvedic treatment I have noted that he tends to analyze the knowledge that he reads critically and tries to apply his understanding of modern medicine and pathology (his field of expertise) to practices traditionally followed in Ayurveda. Starting to self study an entirely different branch of therapeutics may be easy but to persevere and progress in the absence of any help or formal guidance from anyone (especially Ayurvedic fraternity) is all the more difficult and hence very appreciable.

Vast majority of doctors remain busy working in their own area of specialization and they resist deviation from the comfort that this practice provides. There is hardly any inclination to learn and comprehend other systems of medicines with an open mind. To some people this may seem unnecessary and irrelevant but I definitely find this whole exercise of experimenting and writing on the challenging new subject of integrated medicine …. a road less travelled….. unique and innovative. Dr. Amol Sir's work should serve as a source of inspiration for many more to tread this path. That is the reason I have the pleasure to recommend this book to students and researchers of all 3 pathies.

Research into development of therapeutic protocols using integrated medicine approach and the resultant widening of therapeutic armamentarium has the potential to revolutionize medical practice. It will foster more acceptance from doctors of all 3 pathies , bring in respect and credibility to integrated medical practice and help ailing society at large. It could bring an entirely new perspective to integrating healthcare and Dr. Amol has nailed it here.

I congratulate Dr. Amol Javdekar for his very first attempt in writing about a difficult new field and wish him the very best for all his future endeavours.

DR. Poonam Phal B.A.M.S , M.B.A (HCS)

.FOREWORD FROM DR. JYOTI MUNDARGI

Dr. Amol Javdekar was introduced to me by a fellow practitioner during a planning meet on World Cow Medicine Parishad. He told me about his book on integrated medicine which I promptly purchased. I must say it's a very nicely written book – profound in knowledge and easy to understand. Atleast I am not aware of any other book on this topic and also not aware of any pathologist who does clinical practice and that too of all 3 pathies.

Even though Dr. Amol already had basic knowledge of Ayurveda , he telephonically discussed with me his doubts about various treatment regimens in Ayurveda. Even though I have been practising ayurveda for 35 years now and treat a wide variety of diseases from head to toe , I myself learnt many points about various diseases from him which I was not previously aware of. So basically knowledge sharing was two ways in our conversations.

What I found unique about him in all these interactions is his sharp analytical mind and zest to keep on learning. Any single branch of any pathy of medicine is very vast. So I feel even attempting to dwelve into the details of 3 pathies in addition to practising as a pathologist is very commendable.

Another thing worth mentioning is the foresight which Dr. Amol had regarding integrated medicine. He has been studying homeopathy for past 25 years , one year more than his field of specialization that is pathology. So many years back Dr. Amol could predict that the future is of integrated medicine and not only patients even various governments are encouraging research into this intriguing aspect of medical practice.

I felt happy to know that this book has received international recognition and acceptance which it truly deserves and congratulate Dr. Amol for coming out with second edition of this unique book.

Hope even the second edition of this book finds acceptance and appreciation which it truly deserves. My best wishes for that !!

DR. Jyoti Mundargi
B.A.M.S , P.G Diploma in meditation
M.Sc (meditation)

ABOUT THE AUTHOR

Dr. Amol Javdekar is an **alumni of the prestigious B. J. Medical College** – a government medical college attached to Sassoon General Hospitals which is a 1200 bedded hospital.

He completed M.B.B.S in 1997 and M.D (Pathology) in 2002 and has **gold medal in biochemistry and distinction in E.N.T to his credit**. He stood second in Pune University in M.D (Pathology) examination.

During 20 years of post MD work experience , he has worked as a a :

- Lecturer in Miraj Medical College and Bharati Vidyapeeth Medical College , Pune
- Senior Resident in Surgical Pathology in Tata Memorial Hospital and Cancer Research Center , Parel , Mumbai
- Consultant pathologist in Ministry of Health , Kingdom Of Saudi Arabia , Dhande Lab, Pune , Geneombio Technologies Pvt Ltd , Pune and Bliss Diagnostic Center , Pune
- Head of Lab in Lupin Bioresearch Center, Pune , ONP Hospital, Pune and MMDH , Shirur.

Since 2013 he is running his own lab by the name of Goodwill Pathology Lab at Kothrud , Pune – the uniqueness being availability of consultation , path testing and treatment – all in the same place.

Dr. Amol was invited as a speaker in international conference on Bird Flu in Dawadmi General Hospital , K.S.A and on Case Studies in Diabetes in National Conference in Mumbai.

A significant contribution of Dr. Amol Javdekar towards medical education was making of a CD way back in 2007 titled : "3D Animated Medical Teaching Aids " , comprising of around 5000 powerpoint slides and 780 text based pages and covering 34 topics such as Diabetes Mellitus , Acidity , Asthma , Chronic Bronchitis and Emphysema , Thyroid disorders , Obesity , Cirrhosis , Gallstones , PCOD , Melanoma , BEP , Prostate Cancer etc. This CD found its place in the library of some medical colleges and in personal collection of some doctors.

Apart from medical academics , Dr. Amol has many other hobbies such as singing , poem writing and making computer aided designs. He has sung on stage in various functions and has bagged best singer award also. He has written about 20 poems on various topics. He has also designed almost 900 computer aided designs which can be made into frames of 5 different formats and used to decorate home or office.

Contact Details : Mobile : 9822059855

E – mail I.D : dramolj1975@gmail.com

TABLE OF CONTENTS

4. Homeopathy – 41 - 62

- Introduction to Homeopathy
- Principles of Homeopathy
- Homeopathy has a drastically different approach as compared to Allopathy and Ayurveda
- Medicine development and remedy selection in Homeopathy
- Protocols of medicine administration in Homeopathy
- Under what circumstances do patients prefer Homeopathy as primary treatment
- Greatest objections to Homeopathy by non believers
- Why is there so much resistance shown by some patients to take homeopathic treatment
- Advantages of Homeopathy
- Disadvantages / limitations of Homeopathy
- Challenges in front of Homeopathy
- Current state of Homeopathy
- Paradoxical pharmacology – use of Allopathic medicines the homeopathic way
- Choose homeopathy mainly for the following diseases
- A word on biochemic remedies and their comparison with homeopathy
- A word on Bach flower remedies

5. Similarities between the 3 pathies – 63 - 72

- Medicines used in all 3 pathies are sourced from plants , minerals and animals :
- Same medicine may be used by more than one pathy for the same purpose :
- Side effects may be produced by consumption of medicines of all 3 pathies :
- Paralells in theory and practice of Ayurveda and Homeopathy

6. Differences between the 3 pathies – 73 - 85

- Rapidity of onset of action of medicines and speed of cure / control of symptoms
- Predictability of response to treatment
- Dependance liability , rebound effect and its significance in treatment continuation , discontinuation and switching from one pathy to the other
- Tachyphylaxis and drug tolerance

7. Integration of the 3 pathies – 86 - 90

- Why is it essential nowadays to have at least basic understanding of all 3 pathies by practitioners of any pathy ?
- Practice of integrated medicine would pose new challenges

INTRODUCTION

The quest for finding treatments to preserve and restore health is as old as existence of mankind itself.

The history of medicine shows how societies have changed in their approach to illness and disease from ancient times to the present. From crude and painful practices such as blood letting , trepanation and cannibal cures to modern day anesthesia , robotic surgery and prenatal diagnosis medicine has really come a long way.

No one can dispute how medicine has transformed human life and enriched its existence. Thanks to advances in medicine , people are leading longer and more productive lives in spite of stresses of modernism which has negative effect on overall health. Readiness of people to do preventive health check-up and consult doctors at an early stage of disease has yielded rewards in form of better quality of life.

Due to over exposure to easy knowledge available on internet , non medicos , nowadays are aware of numerous alternatives to routine treatment modalities. Some are more than willing to experiment with lesser tested treatment modalities. This attitude has its own rewards and dangers. But the fact remains that people nowadays are more open than ever before to try treatments of all 3 major pathies – Allopathy , Ayurveda and Homeopathy. Cross talk and sharing of experiences between patients further nurtures this trend.

While this makes things easy for patients , it makes life much more complex for the treating doctor who – already overburdened with factual information in his own pathy – has to take additional efforts to know at least basics of the other pathy. Those who don't take the efforts show inclination to deride other pathies in an unfair manner.

Debate about merits and demerits of Allopathy , Ayurveda and Homeopathy is a game of mud slinging with proponents and opponents of each pathy indulging in degrading the other 2 pathies by selectively highlighting only the demerits. Biased opinions are formed after superficial cursory look at responses to treatment by any one pathy rather than after in-depth study of facts by any doctor with reasonably mature knowledge of the pathy to be judged.

Its important to note that the mere fact that all 3 pathies – Allopathy , Ayurveda and Homeopathy – have stood the test of time for hundreds / thousands of years with staunch supporters of them implies that definitely they all have some merits.

And the mere fact that need arose to search for alternative methods to treat various diseases and that there are strong opponents of all 3 pathies implies that definitely they all have some demerits or limitations.

Why waste time , money and energy is just mud slinging? Why not take great efforts to scientifically study all 3 pathies , integrate them , design protocols to improve standards of healthcare and serve humanity in this way.

What I have been doing over past so many years is a humble attempt in this direction.

Doing good quality truthful research , keeping an open mind and unbiased intelligent evaluation of merits and demerits of all 3 pathies are needs of the hour.

This book is written with an aim to introduce and orient the reader to opportunities and challenges in practice of integrated medicine. Aim is certainly not to teach medicine – a much larger book targeted only towards doctors would be needed for that.

Medicine due to its inherent complexity and subjectivity is full of controversies and a relatively new topic like integrated medicine is likely to invite strong criticism. Differences of opinion are bound to be there and it would be wrong to expect every doctor to agree with every point written in this book.

Critical appraisal and suggestions for improving the content of this book are most welcome from doctors and non medicos alike.

-- Dr. Amol Javdekar
M.D (Pathology)

Dear Reader

I am Mother Medicine and this book is my story.

As you can see , I am thousands of year old ….. age has only made me wiser.

I have 3 children - Ayurveda , Allopathy and Homeopathy.

Ayurveda is the oldest - traditional , old fashioned but mature and effective.

Allopathy is my modern "gadget friendly" baccha … smart, intelligent, progressive, quick in giving results and a firm believer in power of evidence.

Homeopathy is my youngest …. thoda hatke hai …. difficult to understand …. very different from the other two …. but magical in results if tapped well..

As a mother , I know all my 3 children have their positives and negatives. It pains me to see them fight with each other all the time. Individually they have so much to offer to the world. They have so much talent in them …. that united… they will achieve the impossible and help me bring smile to each and every ailing mind.

If only they could keep their ego apart……………… try to understand each other and work hand in hand. Hope my 3 children read this story and gain wisdom …for this is as much their story as it is of mine.

Happy Reading !!

AYURVEDA

(Ayur : life ; Veda : science)

INTRODUCTION TO AYURVEDA :

Ayurveda , which literally means science of life and longevity , refers to a 5000 + year old traditional Indian system of medicine based on the idea of balance in bodily systems and uses diet , herbal medicines , yoga , parasurgical and surgical techniques for prevention and treatment of various diseases.

Ayurveda is thus a way of life and is not limited to taking treatment on falling sick but encourages lifestyle changes such that disease can be prevented.

The 3 main treaties of Ayurveda are :

(1) Charaka Samhita : compendium of ancient Indian medicine

(2) Sushrut Samhita : compendium of ancient surgery

(3) Ashtanga Hridaya Samhita : compendium of Indian medicine and surgery.

SALIENT FEATURES OF AYURVEDA :

There are several aspects of this system of medicine which distinguish it from other approaches to health care :

1) Concept of Panchamahabhuta – five great elements from which universe is made

Pancha mahabhutas are five prime elements of nature namely

1) Akash : space / ether

2) Vayu : air

3) Tejas : fire

4) Aapa or Jala : water

5) Prithvi : earth

Ayurveda believes that everything in the universe (including human body) is made from these 5 elements.

2) Concept of Tridoshas :

Tridoshas are bio energies composed of different combinations of 5 basic elements. The 3 doshas – named vata , pitta and kapha - affect all body functions on both mental and physical level. Vata is the dominant one and influences functioning of the other 2 doshas. Good health remains so long as all 3 doshas are in perfect balance. This balance depends on a variety of factors, principally correct diet and exercise, maintaining good digestion, healthy elimination of body wastes and ensuring balanced emotional and spiritual health. Imbalance leads to diseases. During the course of life, the dosha proportions deviate (vikrti) from its original state (prakrti) for various reasons and subsequently, it has an impact on our mental and physical health condition.

1. VATA (air)

Vata biofactor is responsible for functions of the central, autonomic, and peripheral nervous systems. Vata controls the respiratory, blood, lymphatic, excretory, and reproductive systems, as well as all types of movements. It is also responsible for the cognitive functions of the brain, and secretion of various chemical neurotransmitters and hormones.

Identifying vata predominant prakriti :

Thin body , dry , rough skin , dry curly hair , low weak hoarse voice , indecisive , poor memory

Causes of Deranged Vata :

Overworking, grief, worry, lack of sleep, intentional retention of bodily waste, excess exercise or sexual indulgence, and ingestion of bitter, pungent, astringent or dry foods.

Symptoms of Deranged Vata :

Irregular movements (tremors etc) of the limbs, different types of pain , gas problem , contraction of muscles (spasms), roughness / dryness of skin, formation of bone cavities, constipation and an astringent taste in the mouth.

2. PITTA (fire)

It is responsible for appetite, thirst, digestion, metabolism, body heat, normal eyesight, softness of the body, luster, mental calmness, and intelligence. Although pitta , like vata , exists in every cell of the body, the major sites of pitta are believed to be the stomach, duodenum, liver, spleen, pancreas, heart, eyes, and skin.

Identifying pitta predominant prakriti :

Medium height and weight , hot skin , medium size of body parts , strong appetitie , inability to tolerate hunger , hot temper , intelligent , good memory.

Causes of Deranged Pitta :

Pitta may be deranged by ingestion of salty, hot, sharp-tasting foods, as well as by anger. Also by too much planning for future — basically people with lots and lots of ideas.

Symptoms of Deranged Pitta :

Burning sensation in the esophagus and stomach, redness, digestive system disturbances, excessive sweating, fainting, symptoms of intoxication, pungent and sour taste, and inability to see white and dark red color.

3. KAPHA

Kapha is responsible for the normal body moisture, stability of the joints, firmness of the body, a proportionate bulk, weight, strength, endurance, and courage.

Balance of kapha with other humours is function of the lymphatic system, immune system, body fat, and epithelial surfaces with mucous glands.

Kapha balances pitta in functions by providing basic materials for conversion into body tissues by enzymes, a kind of biochemical feedback mechanism. Pitta generates heat from the enzymatic activities, while kapha provides ways to eliminate the heat through the skin, lungs, urine, and faeces via fat and moisture.

Identifying kapha predominant prakriti :

Short , plump or obese , dull , lazy , slow movements , thick moist cold skin , tendency to constipation , slow grasping power but good memory.

Causes of Deranged Kapha :

Overexposure to cold weather; excessive sleep; day sleeping; excessive sweet, fatty, and oily food; low level of physical activity.

Symptoms of Deranged Kapha :

Excess of moisture, bloating of tissues, itching, feeling cold or heavy, low secretory activity, mucous membranes heavily coated with mucous, reduced activity of limbs, swelling, weak digestive power, sleepiness, pale skin, salty taste, and slow recovery after an illness.

Ayurveda believes that so long as these 3 doshas are present in perfect balance health is maintained. Imbalance is the cause of illness.

My comments here are :

(i) there is no objective way to measure quantity of each of these doshas. Ayurvedic doctor is expected to believe in this concept just because its stated in ancient texts.

(ii) Ayurveda accepts that in vast majority of individuals these doshas are present in variable proportions even during relatively healthy states. This makes evaluation of deviation from normal of tridoshas very difficult considering the fact that people come to doctor only when they fall sick thereby not allowing assessment of their own tridosha composition during health.

(iii) whether vitiation of tridoshas during disease is cause or effect of some other underlying pathogenetic mechanism is not clear and how this cause effect relationship is arrived at is also not clear.

To balance the elements and the doshas of the body and mind there are many treatments, therapies, and exercises available.

3) The Sapta Dhatus (seven tissues) :

Ayurveda believes that the human body consists of Sapta dhatus namely :

1. Rasa (tissue fluids)
2. Rakta (blood)
3. Meda (fat and connective tissue)
4. Asthi (bones)
5. Majja (marrow)
6. Mamsa (muscle)
7. Shukra (semen)

These seven tissues work in coordination with each for proper physiological functioning of the human body.

4) The 3 malas (three types of body wastes)

Three types of Body Wastes : viz.-Purisa (faeces),Mutra (urine) and Sveda (sweat).

Ayurveda explains that if the balance between Tridosha is not maintained the waste products of the body are not effectively eliminated and these lead to further complications like diarrhea, constipation, asthma, rheumatoid arthritis and such other complications. If the Mutra Mala (urine) is not removed from the body, it can lead to urinary tract infections, cystitis and gastric pain. If the Sveda Mala is not cleared from the body, it can lead to skin irritation problems, and improper fluid balance.

5) The 3 gunas (satva , rajas and tamas)

The three gunas – Satva ,Rajas and Tamas- are the three essential components or energies of the mind. Ayurveda provides a distinct categorization of people on the basis of their Manasa Prakriti (psychological constitution). Genetically determined, these psychological characteristics are dependent on the relative dominance of the three gunas.

While all individuals have mixed amounts of the three, the predominant guna determines an individual's manasa prakriti. In equilibrium, the three gunas preserve the mind (and indirectly the body), maintaining it in a healthy state. Any disturbance in this equilibrium results in various types of mental disorders.

Satva characterised by lightness , consciousness , pleasure and clarity, is pure, free from disease and cannot be disturbed in any way. It activates the senses and is responsible for the perception of knowledge. Satvik individuals are usually noble and spiritual in character, their nature determined as much by body type as their star constellation, having an element of kapha in their constitution.

Rajas ,the most active of the gunas , has motion and stimulation as its characteristics. All desires , wishes , ambitions and fickle-mindedness are a result of the same. Rajasikas are vulnerable to temptations, are very human in their character and approach to life. Majority of individuals have rajasika bend of mind.

Tamas is characterised by heaviness and resistance. It produces disturbances in the process of perception and activities of the mind. Delusion , false knowledge , laziness , apathy, sleep and drowsiness are due to it.

My comments here are :
(i) environment and upbringing (sanskaras) influence mentality and personality of a person right from the day he / she is born or even by "garbhasanskara " - experiences of mother while baby is still in womb. On what basis does Ayurveda differentiate variable influences of so called genetical from environmental influences on shaping predominant guna of a person is not clear.
(ii) How does Ayurvedic physician -- who sees patient during diseased state and for a very very short span of few minutes to few hours / days -- reliably come to understand guna of patient in such a short time ?
(iii) People tend to behave differently in different situations , with different people and at various stages of life . Is this important factor considered while judging manas prakriti ?

APPROACH TO DISEASE DIAGNOSIS IN AYURVEDA :
Ayurveda has eight ways to diagnose illness. They include :-
1) Nadi pariksha (examination of pulse) : some Ayurvedic physicians are so good in this skill that with very little if any information from patient they can correctly diagnose disease just by pulse examination.

2) Mutra pariksha (examination of urine) : this is somewhat similar to gross examination of urine in modern pathology laboratories. However , compared to the extent of testing that can be done on urine – gross , chemical , microscopic and various others in special cases – urine examination information as mentioned in ancient Ayurvedic texts is very limited and describes but a very few diseases. Further since modern day microscopes were not available in the ancient times when Ayurveda was developed there is no mention about microscopic urine findings in various diseases.

3) Purisha pariksha (examination of stool) : After digestion, the Sarabhaga (nutrient portion) gets absorbed and the remaining undigested part becomes solid and that is called as Purisha. The changes pertaining to Purisha (stool) have been described under various disease conditions in Brihattrayi but are scattered. In Ayurvedic texts, examination of stool is limited mainly up to the examination of physical characteristics such as color, quantity, odor, froth, and consistency. Besides these, a specialized technique of stool examination, i.e., Jala Nimajjana Purisha Pariksha has been described to detect the presence of Ama thereby inferring the status of Agni in the body. Characteristics of normal stool in terms of physical characteristics are not described separately in the ancient and medieval period texts of Ayurveda.

4) Jivha pariksha (examination of tongue): Various features of the tongue are examined such as shape, colour, moisture, movement and the coating on the tongue. Jivha pariksha reveals our main constitution (normal prakruti), imbalance of doshas, state of agni (digestive fire) and koshtha (Annavaha strotas). According to Ayurveda Agnimandya (hypo functioning of digestive fire) is the root cause of all diseases. Saam jivha (white coated tongue) indicates a presence of ama (undigested   food) in the digestive system. Thick coating indicates the progression of disease.

--- ≈≈≈≈≈≈ ◉ Multi – Pathy Co – relation ◉ ≈≈≈≈≈≈ ---

It is interesting to note here that examination of tongue is given importance in Allopathy also and characteristics of tongue plays an important role in remedy selection in Homeopathy. For example thick white coat on tongue is a pointer to use of ***antim crud*** whereas clean tongue in a patient with nausea and vomiting is a pointer to use of ***ipecac*** in Homeopathy.

5) Shabda pariksha (speech) : The person's ability or strength to speak, continuity of thought , hoarseness etc, can hint about diseases pertaining to speech centers in brain and vocal apparatus as well as give idea about overall intellect and level of education of patient.

6) Sparsha (touch) pariksha : This is somewhat similar to palpation method of clinical assessment which is part of modern medicine clinical examination.

7) Druk (vision) pariksha : Assessment of vision : Apart from visual acuity , examination of eye as such is also done in Ayurveda noting color of sclera, conjuctiva, size of eye ball, dryness, shape, area around eyes etc.

8) Aakruti pariksha (appearance) : The overall appearance of patient – body frame , proportion of body parts , outwardly visible physical features provides valuable information about vata – pitta – kapha body type composition as well as educational , intellectual level and mental status and nature of patient.

Although akriti pariksha / appearance has limited role in disease diagnosis or remedy selection in modern medicine , in Homeopathy , while selecting constitutional homeopathic medicines physical appearance plays an important role. Thus for example , calcarea carb is found to help fat , flabby , round contoured patients more when compared to phosphorus which is found to help tall , thin , narrow chested patients.

APPROACH OF AYURVEDIC TREATMENT :

The first step in Ayurvedic management of any illness is searching for faults in patients heredity , diet and lifestyle with an aim to rectify them. The causative factors must be stopped in order to slow down the disease process. Thus for example , if a person is suffering from severe acidity due to wrong eating habits and hectic stressful lifestyle , diet and lifestyle needs to be changed rather than just giving ayurvedic medicines to control acidity. After giving sufficient time for healing process to begin with above measures , improvement can be speeded by administration of ayurvedic herbs and making use of some therapeutic techniques like panchakarma.

Herbs and treatments are given based on a thorough analysis of the health condition. The above are aimed at removing weakness (dhatu daurbalya) which allowed disease to begin in first place and actually negative the dosha imbalance.

Ayurveda recognizes the unique constitutional differences of all individuals and therefore recommends different treatments for different types of people. Although two people may appear to have the same outward symptoms, their energetic constitutions may be very different and therefore call for very different remedies.

Thus it would be wrong for general public to self treat based on information available on internet , whattsapp messages etc.

Coming back to treatment modalities available in Ayurveda :

Management of illness primarily consists of four procedures:

(1) cleansing (samsodhan),

(2) palliation (Shamana)

(3) rejuvenation (kaya kalp)

(4) mental and spiritual healing (sattvavajaya, or psychotherapy).

(1) Cleansing : The major cause of body ailments is the toxic products produced by body metabolism, microorganisms, synthetic chemicals, xenobiotics or drugs.
The management of an illness starts with cleansing and includes five procedures called **PANCHAKARMA**. Panchakarma includes :

Vamana : induction of vomiting to balance kapha and pitta doshas In diseases like sinusitis bronchitis , asthma , skin diseases resulting form kapha pitta imbalance.

Virechana : induction of loose motions to reduce pitta excess – esp useful in hyperacidity , urticaria , herpes etc.

Basti : Rectal administration of medicated oils etc to reduce vata dosha seen in backache , arthritis , multiple sclerosis etc.

Raktamoshana : removing unhealthy blood from body using leeches , scalp vein set which may provide instant relief in diseases like migraine , piles , abscess , arthritis , toothache , acute appendicitis

Nasya : Instillation into nose of medicated oil drops useful for all diseases above clavicle.

(2) Palliation : Palliation essentially consists of use of compound preparations of herbs and minerals for diet and lifestyle interventions.
Ayurvedic texts describe seven types of palliation:

      (1) digestive power enhancement
      (2) toxic waste (ama) elimination
      (3) fasting,
      (4) observing thirst
      (5) yoga exercise
      (6) lying in the sunlight or sunbathing
      (7) breathing exercise and meditation.

(3) Rejuvenation (kaya kalp) : Rasayana or rejuvenation is a traditional Ayurvedic therapy to restore the body's vitality to its fullest capacity using herbs and procedures bestows youthfulness and cures disease. If taken in a proper way, Rasayana helps maintain youthfulness and keeps you fit both physically and mentally for many years. In the Rasayana treatments individual is given guidance to properly withdraw from sensory stimuli like Shabda (sound), Sparsha (touch), Roopa (visuals), Rasa (unwanted taste) and Gandha (unpleasant smell). Thereby mind gets gradually withdrawn from sensory subjects and gets aligned with pranic level. In this period, timely practice of pranayama, mudra and chantings improve flow of prana through nadis (channels of prana) and chakras. Along with this, balanced and nourishing diet, rasayana medicines regenerates new cells in the body. Formation of new cells and existence of healthier cells improves tissue level health and thereby establishes ojus. Rasayana therapy is indicated for people suffering from the following problems or illnesses : stress, insomnia, shallow breath, rough and dry skin, weak senses and sexual strength, weak appetite, lack of concentration, weak memory, chronic digestive problems, constipation, migraine and obesity. It should be taken for minimum 21 days and for better result for 4 to 6 weeks.

Depending on health status at time of consultation , proper guidance will be given by the Ayurveda doctor, based on assessment.

(4) mental and spiritual healing (sattvavajaya, or psychotherapy) : Satvavajaya Chikitsa (Ayurvedic psychotherapy) is a nonpharmacological approach aimed at control of mind and restraining it from unwholesome Artha (objects) or stressors. Withdrawal of the mind from unwholesome objects is known as Sattvavajaya Chikitsa or it is a treatment by Self Control. Thus, it includes all the methods of Manonigraha and Astanga Yoga (Yogic techniques) too. Indian philosophy portrays Astanga Yoga as a primary tool to control mind; hence it can be used as Satvavajaya Chikitsa.

CHOOSE AYURVEDA MAINLY FOR THE FOLLOWING :
1) Allergies : rhinitis , asthma , atopic dermatitis
2) Psychological problems : anxiety , depression , insanity
3) Arthritis : rheumatoid , gouty
4) Back pain , sciatica
5) Bronchitis
6) Varicose veins
7) Colds and chronic cough
8) Digestive complaints such as IBS , constipation , indigestion , diarrhoea
9) Urological problems : urine hesitancy , polyuria , incontinence etc
10) Neurological issues : paralysis , nerve palsies
11) Headaches
12) High blood pressure
13) Insomnia
14) Liver disorders
15) Female and male reproductive issues including infertility
16) Skin problems : eczema , psoriasis

HOW EFFECTIVE IS AYURVEDA IN TREATMENT OF EMERGENCY CONDITIONS ? :

The general opinion of lay public , non ayurvedic doctors and even some Ayurvedic doctors is : Ayurveda is very slow to act and has nothing to offer in medical emergencies. Honestly I admit that even I had the same opinion about Ayurveda till a few months ago when further studies and interaction with Ayurvedic experts changed my view.

There are certain ayurvedic parasurgical techniques like Viddha karma , Agni karma which are known to show amazing results within seconds.

Viddha karma includes insertion of very fine hollow needles into certain specific points of the body to produce desired therapeutic benefit.

Agnikarma involves momentary application of heat to skin surface using special needles (shallakas) of various metals. **Judicious use of above 2 techniques in acute conditions like severe abdominal pain due to ureteric colic , menstrual cramps , acute onset breathlessness due to asthma , conditions like anosmia , ageusia etc. can produce results within seconds to minutes.**

Pradhaman nasya using vacha shunthi combination can awaken an unconscious patient within seconds.

Basti when used judiciously can remove all sorts of pains within minutes to hours. Raktamokshan has the power to reduce pain due to vitiated rakta (vatarakta or raktapitta) even before the procedure is complete.

The exact details of above procedures is beyond the scope of discussion of this book.

<u>Even life threatening conditions like acute myocardial infarction and stroke can be helped by emergency ayurvedic procedures.</u>

Ayurvedic treatment can even be used as a complimentary treatment within I.C.U. But it is important that this be done by expert vaidyas who should be allowed to do so by modern medicine doctors.

ROLE OF WESTERN MODERN MEDICAL TREATMENT AND AYURVEDIC TREATMENT IN HEALTHCARE :

Both Western modern medicine and Ayurveda are based on the principle of **CONTRARIA CONTRARIS CURANTUR** (LATIN) which means opposites are cured by opposites. This principle teaches to treat disease by using remedies that produce opposite effects. Thus acidity is treated by using acid nullifying alkaline chemicals in modern medicine and herbs with antacid effects in ayurveda. Homeopathy , on the other hand is based on the principle : SIMILIA SIMILIBUS CURANTUR.

The principles of Ayurvedic treatment are for the most part the same as those of allopathic treatment. They consist of removing the injurious agent, soothing the injured body and mind, and eradicating the cause. The difference lies in the methods adopted by the two systems.

All Ayurvedic doctors are taught modern anatomy , physiology and biochemistry in their first year BAMS curriculum. Ayurvedic theoretical concepts regarding etiopathogenesis and disease pathophysiology are taught later on. According to expert Ayurvedic vaidyas problem arises when Ayurvedic doctors take modern medicine approach to disease diagnosis and treat using ayurveda. Example : although modern Ayurvedic doctors read and try to understand modern anatomy -- drawing exact parallels between circulatory system anatomy and strotas in ayurveda is wrong according to them.

HOW CAN AYURVEDA BE INTEGRATED INTO MODERN MEDICAL PRACTICE :
This is actually already being done especially when it comes to administration of ayurvedic hepatoprotective medicines (LIV 52 etc) by allopathic doctors. In Allopathy , there are almost no highly effective medicines for terminal liver disease of a non neoplastic etiology. This is one area where Ayurveda exhibits superiority to modern medicine because of availability of highly effective medicines to treat above mentioned diseases.

Allopathic hepatoprotective drugs , synthesized in lab exhibit minimal effectiveness in improving liver cell mass and reversing the damage done. Moreover the side effects and the drug interactions are major restrictions in their clinical utility. On the other hand, herbal medicines are widely used across the globe due to their wide applicability and therapeutic efficacy coupled with least side effects. Garden nightshade , chicory , lettuce , blackberry , fumaria , coffee, senna , aloe vera , celery , grapewine etc have proven hepatoprotective effects.

As far as renal failure is concerned , at stage 3 and stage 4 chronic kidney disease , irrespective of what proponents of Ayurveda and Homeopathy might claim , close scrutiny reveals that for vast majority of patients dialysis or renal transplant offers the best and most reliable cure currently available. Studies of Ayurvedic medicines done on stage 1 and stage 2 chronic kidney disease are of poor quality and reveal contradictory information. Benefits shown in these studies using exclusive Ayurvedic medicines are very unimpressive and limited.

PERSONALIZED MEDICINE :

Personalized medicine (individualized medicine) is defined as medical care for each patient's unique condition. Out of the 3 pathies , homeopathy shows individualization in medicine selection to an extreme degree. Individualization is less in Ayurveda and even lesser in Alllopathy.

Father of western medicine, Hippocrates was also known to advocate personalized medicine. He evaluated factors like person's constitution, age and physique in decision making when prescribing drugs.

In the 21st century, personalized medicine is all about utilizing knowledge of genetic make up of a patient related to drug pharmacokinetics and pharmacodynamics to give patient specific treatment.

Pharmacogenomics is the foundation to personalized healthcare. Pharmacogenomics analyzes how the genetic makeup of an individual affects his/her response to drugs. Diet, overall health, and environment also have significant influence on medication response, but genetic make up is the strongest influence of response to medication.

Knowledge of pharmacogenomics helps in following ways :
(1) Improve drug safety and reduce adverse drug reactions
(2) Tailor treatments to match patients' unique genetic pre-disposition
(3) Identify optimal dose of any medicine
(4) Improve drug discovery targeted to human disease and
(5) Improve proof of principle for efficacy trials.

Pharmacogenomics may be applied to several areas of medicine, including pain management, cardiology, oncology, and psychiatry.
In cancer treatment, pharmacogenomics tests are used to identify which patients are most likely to respond to certain cancer drugs.

Although knowledge of genetics was not available thousands of years ago when foundations of Ayurveda were being laid down , by keen observation Ayurvedic physicians were able to put forth the tridosha theory which forms the basis of Prakriti-based medicine. Each 'Prakriti' has varying degree of predisposition to different diseases.

<u>Ayurgenomics is the integration of the principles of Ayurveda with genomics.</u> The primary challenge of Ayurgenomics is to establish the correlation between DNA and 'Prakriti'. The basis of individual variations in Ayurveda indicates that individuals with Pitta Prakriti are fast metabolizers while those of Kapha Prakriti are slow metabolizers. Different prakriti may have different drug metabolism rates associated with drug etabolizing enzyme (DME) polymorphism as well. A correlation between CYP2C19 enzymes involved in metabolism of a number of drugs genotypes and prakriti has been studied. Therefore Ayurgenomics seems to bear similarities with pharmacogenetics and has the potential to be a platform to achieve personalized drug therapy. The understanding of "SNP science – Single Nucleotide Polymorphism science " lead to the concept of personalized medicine which goes parallel with the concept of "Prakriti based medicine (Ayurgenomics)."

CONCLUDING REMARKS :
Ayurveda is a unique traditional Indian system of medicine which emphasizes life style intervention , dietary regulation etc along with medicines for prevention and treatment of diseases. In addition it has its own parasurgical and surgical techniques.

Its role is mainly in treatment of chronic degenerative or life style related diseases. Having said that scores of expert Ayurvedic vaidyas have successfully used pure ayurveda in handling medical emergencies with very good results.

Modernism is slowly entering Ayurvedic practice with modification of various instruments used for Panchakarma procedures etc. Its good to see research papers published to refute or confirm age old Ayurvedic knowledge as well as to add to it.

It's a myth that ayurvedic treatment is not associated with side effects. Side effects certainly do occur if ayurvedic medicines are used improperly – because of half knowledge or total lack of knowledge regarding their correct use.

In the days to come Ayurveda has bright future and is likely to become modality of choice atleast in treatment of some diseases.

ALLOPATHY

(Allos : other ; Pathos : suffering)

INTRODUCTION TO ALLOPATHY :

Allopathy refers to evidence based modern medicine evolved on strong foundations of basic sciences and spectacular advances in applied medical streams . The term Allopathy which means " other suffering " is a derogatory term coined by 19th century homeopathic physicians to refer to heroic medical practices present at that time which subjected patient to tremendous pain and employed measures for which there was no evidence. Such heroic practices included repeated bloodletting , purgation and induced sweating and were very troublesome to the patients with poor benefits if any.

Since the Allopathy practised today is totally different from that practised more than 200 years ago and because it was a derogatory term when first used many modern day physicians object to its usage and **prefer to use the word modern medicine which is evidence based medicine (EBM) .**
This is indeed agreeable and acceptable because no other pathy has scientifically progressed and shown improvements in treatment protocols as has Allopathy or modern medicine.

Alas , misnomers are deeply entrenched in medical science and very reluctantly we continue use of word Allopathy simply because its well known to all.

Modern medicine, or medicine as we know it, started to emerge after the Industrial Revolution in the 18th century. At this time, there was rapid growth in economic activity in Western Europe and the Americas.

During the 19th century, scientists made rapid progress in identifying and preventing illnesses and highly effective , predictable and reproducible treatment protocols came into existence thanks to advances in basic sciences of anatomy , physiology , biochemistry , pathology , microbiology and pharmacology.

SIGNIFICANT CONTRIBUTIONS OF ALLOPATHY / MODERN MEDICINE TO HUMANITY :

(1) Vaccines : Throughout the 1800s and early 1900s, various vaccinations were created to combat some of the world's deadliest diseases, including smallpox, rabies, tuberculosis, and cholera. Over the course of 200 years, one of the deadliest diseases known to man – the small pox – was wiped off the face of the earth. Today, vaccines continue to save millions of lives each year – preventing diseases such as the deadly flu , tuberculosis , tetanus , H. Influenza meningitis , Hepatitis – B etc .

(2) Anesthesia : Before the first use of a general anaesthetic in the mid-19th century, surgery was undertaken only as a last resort, with several patients opting for death rather than enduring the excruciating pain of surgery. William T. G. Morton made history in 1846 when he successfully used ether as an anaesthetic during surgery. Over the 150 years since, safer anaesthetics have been developed, allowing millions of life-saving, painless operations to take place.

(3) Germ Theory : Before the 'germ' theory came about, the widely believed theory was that disease was caused by 'spontaneous generation'. In other words, physicians of the time thought that disease could appear out of thin air, rather than being air-borne or transferred via skin-to-skin contact. In 1861, French microbiologist Louis Pasteur proved through a simple experiment that infectious disease was a result of an invasion of specific microscopic organisms - also known as pathogens - into living hosts. This new understanding marked a significant turning point in how diseases were treated, controlled and prevented, helping to prevent devastating epidemics that were responsible for thousands of deaths every year, such as the plague, dysentery and typhoid fever.

(4) Medical imaging : The first medical imaging machines were X-rays invented in 1895 by German physicist Wilhelm Conrad Röntgen when experimenting with electrical currents through glass cathode-ray tubes. The discovery transformed medicine overnight and by the following year, Glasgow hospital opened the world's very first radiology department.

Ultrasound , which entered medical diagnosis in 1955 , was a ground-breaking advancement helping detect thoracic , abdominal , prenatal and soft tissue abnormalities.
In 1967, the computed tomography (CT) scanner was created, which uses X-ray detectors and computers to diagnose many different types of disease, and has become a fundamental diagnostic tool in modern medicine.

The next major medical imaging technology was MRI - discovered in 1973 . The nuclear magnetic resonance data creates detailed images within the body and is a crucial tool in detecting life-threatening conditions including tumours, cysts, damage to the brain and spinal cord and some heart and liver problems.

(5) Antibiotics : Alexander Fleming's penicillin, the world's first antibiotic, completely revolutionised the war against deadly bacteria. For many years antibiotics served as the feather in crown of modern medicine by predictably and reliably reducing disease symptoms caused by bacteria susceptible to the antibiotic. Unfortunately, over the years some bacteria have become increasingly resistant to antibiotics, leading to a world-wide crisis that calls for the pharmaceutical industry to develop new anti-bacterial treatments as soon as possible.

(6) Anti – viral drugs : Terrible viruses such as small-pox, influenza and hepatitis have ravaged many human populations throughout history. The development of effective antivirals has been significant in treating and controlling the spread of deadly virus outbreaks such as HIV/AIDS, Ebola and rabies.

(7) Organ transplant : In December 1954, the first successful kidney transplant was carried out by Dr Joseph Murray and Dr David Hume in Boston, USA. Technical developments in vascular anastomosis , surgical techniques of organ placement and ability to control rejection which is immune response by recipients body paved way for increasing success of organ transplants . In 1963, the first lung transplant was carried out, followed by a pancreas/kidney in 1966, and liver and heart in 1967. Aside from saving thousands of lives in the years following, transplant procedures have also become increasingly innovative and complex, with doctors successfully completing the first hand transplant in 1998 and full-face transplant in 2010.

(8) Stem cell therapy : The incredible potential of stem cells was discovered in the late 1970s, when they were found inside human cord blood. Two specific characteristics make stem cells remarkable: they are unspecialised cells that can renew themselves through cell division even after being inactive, and under certain conditions can be used to make any type of human cell. This discovery has enormous potential and stem cell therapy has already been used to treat leukaemia and other blood disorders, as well as in bone marrow transplantation. Research is currently ongoing to use stem cells to treat spinal cord injuries and a number of neurological conditions such as Alzheimer's, Parkinson' and strokes. However many ethical issues need to be addressed to prevent its misuse.

(9) Immunotherapy : Immunotherapy, a treatment that stimulates the immune system to fight off a disease, has been in the making for over a century. The story began in the 1890s with the experimental work of William B. Coley who injected inactive bacteria into cancerous tumours, achieving remission in some patients. However, it is only in the last 40 years that serious progress has been made in immunotherapy, particularly in respect to treating cancer. In the 1970s, antibody therapies were developed and in 1991, researchers produced the first cancer vaccine which was approved by the FDA in 2010. In the last decade, immuno-oncology has become one of the most revolutionary cancer therapies in existence.

<u>Modern medicine has offered really a lot to mankind and this is a byproduct of centuries of extreme hardwork by brilliant doctors and scientists who have used their intelligence for the betterment of mankind. They deserve the greatest possible respect and gratitude from all of us.</u>

PRINCIPLES OF ALLOPATHY :
(1) Make a proper diagnosis before initiating treatment :
Modern medical practice rests on the premise that treatment of any patient should always follow and be based on a correct diagnosis. That is to say , shooting bullets (treatment) in pitch darkness with the hope that at least one bullet will hit the target (cure / control the disease) is not considered rational modern medical practice.
Correct diagnosis begins with a thorough history and proper clinical examination. Pathology and radiology tests are done to confirm or refute differential diagnosis that forms in clinician's mind at end of clinical evaluation. Spectacular advancements in both these diagnostic branches have made it almost imperative that a sound diagnosis be made before treatment is started.

Note here that there are other uses of pathology and radiology tests beyond establishing diagnosis such as :
- evaluation of kidney and liver functioning before giving certain medicines
- evaluation for vitamin deficiencies which need to be rectified for optimum treatment
- evaluation of extent of a particular disease

- prognostication : giving idea to patient about chances of survival or chances of living with morbidity

Thus pathologists and radiologists are playing increasingly important roles in overall patient management.

I want to emphasize this point to non medico readers of this book that **when treating doctor advices them to do certain tests please do not always view this act with suspicion.** If the doctor explains the need – go ahead and do the test. Don't pressurize your doctor to start treatment before proper diagnosis is done. Doctors often reluctantly start treatment hurriedly because of previous bad experience with other patients who leave them when asked to do some tests.

(2) Drugs which show distinct statistically significant advantage over placebo in RCTs (Randomized Control Trials) only should be accepted as medicine.

A randomized control trial or RCT is a scientific medical experiment that aims to reduce certain sources of bias when testing the effectiveness of new treatments ; this is accomplished by randomly allocating subjects to two or more groups, treating them differently, and then comparing them with respect to a measured response.

One group—the experimental group—receives the intervention being assessed, while the other—usually called the control group—receives an alternative treatment, such as a placebo or no intervention. The groups are monitored under conditions of the trial design to determine the effectiveness of the experimental intervention, and efficacy is assessed in comparison to the control.

The trial may be blinded, meaning that information which may influence the participants is withheld until after the experiment is complete. A blind can be imposed on any participant of an experiment, including subjects, researchers, technicians, data analysts, and evaluators. Effective blinding may reduce or eliminate some sources of experimental bias.

The randomness in the assignment of subjects to groups reduces selection bias. Blinding reduces other forms of experimenter and subject biases.

A well-blinded RCT is often considered the gold standard for clinical trials. Blinded RCTs are commonly used to test the efficacy of medical interventions and may additionally provide information about adverse effects, such as drug reactions. Before any medicine or other treatment modality gets accepted it has to pass this scrutiny.

(3) Scrutiny by peer review : Importance of evidence based medicine

In modern day practice of Allopathy , before any treatment modality or protocol (medical / surgical , mixed) gets accepted it is **mandatory for researchers to publish their findings regarding usage of the treatment in reputed peer reviewed journals so that they are scrutinized by other experts in the field before being accepted or rejected**. Its not easy to falsify findings and get away with it because competing groups of researchers have the liberty to carry out exact same research to cross verify and see if they get the same results or not. **Just research is not sufficient , quality of research is also important – methodology , sample size , confounding factors , inferences etc etc.**

Thus one has to furnish strong irrefutable evidence before taking credit for devising a new treatment strategy. Hence modern medicine is nowadays referred to as "evidence based medicine or EBM ". Evidence-based medicine (EBM) is "the conscientious, explicit and judicious use of current best evidence in making decisions about the care of individual patients." The aim of EBM is to integrate the experience of the clinician, the values of the patient, and the best available scientific information to guide decision-making about clinical management. The term was originally used to describe an approach to teaching the practice of medicine and improving decisions by individual physicians about individual patients.

Its not that research is not carried out in Ayurveda and Homeopathy but the quality of research for the majority of times is of very poor quality and has no value as far as its reliability is concerned. Lack of adequate high caliber research continues to be major drawback of Ayurveda and Homeopathy till this day. ***Please note here that I am referring to lack of adequacy and not to non existence of high caliber research.*** This does not mean Ayurvedic and homeopathic treatments are useless or of inferior quality – what is means is there is inadequate evidence to support their usage for treating various disease conditions. By inadequate evidence I mean documented evidence – not hearsay anecdotal evidence. Considering how much Ayurvedic and Homeopathic medicine manufacturers are profiting from sale of their medicine these days , its difficult to understand why part of the profits cant be reinvested in studying the medicines in a better way.

ALLOPATHY IS THE UNEQUIVOCAL LEADER WHEN IT COMES TO DIAGNOSTICS , SURGICAL ADVANCES AND MANAGEMENT OF ACUTE EMERGENCIES :

Advances in pathology and radiology has revolutionized disease diagnosis. This has helped tremendously in understanding various disease processes which may have same symptoms outwardly but totally different mechanisms underlying their production. In depth understanding of pathogenetic mechanisms has provided ideas to treatment developments. High tech diagnostic machinery has brought reliability and reproducibility to disease diagnosis – something which didn't exist as recent as 3 to 4 decades ago. Its now possible to give irrefutable evidence of causes of certain diseases which negative critics of Allopathy (usually doctors of Ayurveda and Homeopathy) can just not disregard.

Example 1 : Patient comes with signs and symptoms suggestive of - say – bacterial infection of oropharynx and tonsils – oropharyngeal swab is sent to pathology lab for culture which reports growth of gram positive bacteria . Physician gives antibiotics and other symptomatic treatment , patient gets relief from all his suffering. Repeat swab from same area now yields no growth. See the logic of approach ? Such is the level of logic and clarity in Allopathic practice. Who can refute such rock solid evidence ?

Example 2 : Patient presents with fits of loud sneezing on getting exposed to dust and develops runny nose , headache and nasopharyngeal itching. Treating doctor suspects allergic rhinitis , asks for hemogram and serum total IgE. Reports show eosinophilia and raised serum total IgE levels. Antihistaminics , steroids , mast cell stabilizers etc are given , patients gets tremendous relief from all his symptoms. After few days of complete recovery , hemogram done shows normal eosinophil counts and normal serum total IgE levels. Once again – scientifically acceptable chain of events – leading to predictability of results.

Example 3 : Patient comes with signs and symptoms suggestive of deficiencies of iron , vitamin B 12 , vitamin D etc . The actual deficiency is confirmed by pathology lab tests - supplements given to remove the deficiency - patient starts feeling better and better and repeat testing confirms normalization of values.

Example 4 : Patient comes with fever , productive cough with chest pain during coughing , expectoration of rusty sputum. Pneumonia is suspected and confirmed by chest X ray or CT scan. CRP is raised , one specific organism is grown on sputum culture. Antibiotics given as per culture sensitivity report relieves the patient from all symptoms and he / she feels distinctly better. Repeat testing of all abnormal tests confirm normalization of values and findings.

There are many more examples , where Allopathy is the best pathy as far as understanding of disease processes in scientifically acceptable terms is concerned.

Not only are non medicos impressed with this concreteness of Allopathy but very routinely in clinical practice , Ayurvedic and homeopathic doctors take help of modern diagnostic modalities like pathology and radiology to understand what is going wrong in their patients. Once proper diagnosis is made , further treatment changes depending on whether patient is going to be treated with Allopathy , Ayurvedic or homeopathic or mixed treatment.

Similarly , there have been such spectacular improvements in surgical procedures in modern medicine like cataract surgery , total knee replacement , bariatric surgery for morbidly obese patients that I would always advice my patients to give first preference to surgical treatment if suffering from any of the above diseases.

While writing first edition of this book I was under the wrong impression that Ayurveda has nothing to offer to treatment of medical emergencies. I knew that modern medicine leads the way in management of numerous acute or emergency conditions. Was also aware that homeopathy has the potential to be used successfully in medical emergencies. However , as I have mentioned before , I now know that Ayurveda also has a lot to offer in treatment of medical emergencies and can be combined with other 2 pathies.

ALLOPATHY FALLS SHORT IN TREATMENT OF SOME CHRONIC AILMENTS AND SOME PECULIAR HEALTH ISSUES OF PATIENT :

When it comes to treatment of liver diseases , many types of neurological medical diseases , some common diseases like chronic sinusitis , various autoimmune or rheumatic problems like rheumatoid arthritis , SLE , psoriasis , behavioral disorders , treatment of some viral diseases Allopathy falls short of expectations. Allopathic treatment of some of these diseases is at times purely symptomatic and does not address the root cause at all. At times results are suboptimal and at other times poor patient is subjected to horrifying side effects resulting from long term consumption of medicines.

Ayurveda leads the way in management of many life style related chronic diseases because of superior results of treatment.

On the other hand , **Homeopathy and only Homeopathy has the solution** to sufferings at very early stages of some diseases when proper diagnosis is difficult or not possible. Patient is suffering but when they ask Allopathic or Ayurvedic doctors what is the diagnosis no answer can be given. At such early stages in disease evolution patient may exhibit PQRS (peculiar , queer , rare and strange) symptoms / signs. If patient correctly describes these PQRS symptoms and homeopath correctly administers the true similimum patient's health is restored to normal with minimum cost and almost no side effects.

WHAT IRKS SOME PATIENTS ABOUT ALLOPATHY AND DRIVES THEM TO SEEK TREATMENT FROM PRACTITIONERS OF OTHER PATHIES :

One of the most common and acceptable complaints of patients especially against Allopathic doctors is that they do not give sufficient time , do not ask anything about diet , life style and sleep and prescribe medicine in shortest possible time in a very mechanistic fashion. Not all object to this , but those who find such an attitude of the doctor objectionable report high satisfaction after visiting an Ayurvedic or Homeopathic doctor who spends much more time with the patient. **Its worthwhile to note here that this objection has nothing to do with Allopathy or modern medicine as a science but with the way it is practised.**

The other thing which bothers some patients is the numerous medicines that are prescribed for each of the different health issue. Thus for example , where an Allopathic doctor may prescribe a different medicine each for diabetes mellitus , hypertension , acidity , asthma , joint pains and insomnia (totalling 6 or more medicines) for one patient , a classic homeopath would attempt to find just one medicine that would stimulate patient's vital force and help bring about an overall improvement in person's health.

An Ayurvedic doctor would also use a more limited number of medicines but here I want to point out a very important fact. **Majority of the fixed dose Ayurvedic medicines prescribed to patients may appear to be one medicine to the patient but in fact are a combination of more than 20 herbs mixed in specific manner.** Thus it would be wrong if the Ayurvedic doctor claims to have given the patient just one medicine when in fact that one medicine contains numerous ingredients.

WHY IS IT IMPORTANT TO KEEP NUMBER OF MEDICINES USED TO A MINIMUM:
There are 4 main reasons why every attempt should be made by treating doctor to keep number of medicines to bare minimum.
Reason 1 : Cost factor : As number of medicines increase cost of treatment increases and for majority of patients long term over spending on health is not possible.

Reason 2 : Side effects : Medicines of all 3 pathies may be associated with side effects – which are nothing but actions of medicines that are undesirable. At times it so happens that as medicine use is continued side effects which appeared at beginning of treatment may wane off and beneficial health effects remain forever. Example is long term use of Metformin for treatment of diabetes mellitus. Some patients may experience side effects like metallic taste , vague abdominal pain in the beginning of treatment. But with some adjustments told by treating doctor and prolonged use these side effects disappear and beneficial effects on blood sugar remain.

On the other hand with some medicines , side effects appear only after prolonged use of the medicines. Thus in Ayurveda side effects occur only after prolonged non stop use of rejuvenators like Triphala , Shatavari , Vidarikanda etc.

Reason 3 : Drug interactions : When more than one medicine is used they interact with each to produce beneficial or harmful effects. The chances that adverse drug reactions (ADR) would occur rises with the number of drugs used.

Beneficial effects are harnessed by making fixed dose combinations (FDCs) of drugs / medicines. For example : vitamin C is added to iron preparations to increase absorption of iron. When carbidopa is added to levodopa in treatment of Parkinsonism , the dose of Levodopa can be reduced as much as 75% and side effects such as nausea , vomiting , palpitations , postural hypotension can be prevented.

Side effect of one drug can be nullified by effect of other drug. For example constipating effect of aluminium hydroxide is countered by laxative effect of magnesium trisilicate when they are combined with each other as a FDC antacid.

Similarly soporific effects of Chlorpheniramine maleate are countered by stimulant effects of phenylephrine when they are combined with each other as FDC anti cold medicine.

With the same logic many proprietary Ayurvedic medicines have numerous ingredients which have been combined because they cancel side effects of each other or promote absorption of other ingredients.

However , when multiple single medicines are used to help control different diseases in same patient following problems can occur :

(1) Interference with absorption :
- Calcium , magnesium , aluminium and iron salts interfere with absorption of tetracycline and of prednisolone
- Sucralfate reduces bioavailability of phenytoin

- Sodium bicarbonate elevates gastric pH and reduces absorption of tetracycline
- Anti muscarinic drugs and opioids can slow down the absorption of other drugs by delaying gastric emptying

(2) Interference with drug distribution :

- Clofibrate can displace warfarin sodium from protein bindings sites increasing blood levels of free warfarin leading to bleeding tendency
- Salicylates can displace glibenclamide from protein binding sites increasing blood levels of free glibenclamide leading to hypoglycemia

(3) Interference with drug transport :

Guanethidine and reserpine which are adrenergic neurone blocking drugs are actively transported into adrenergic neuron by the same transport system that is responsible for noradrenaline uptake into the neuron. This system is inhibited by the anti depressant imipramine which interferes with the antihypertensive activity of guanethidine / reserpine.

(4) Interference with drug metabolism :

- Stimulation : The synthesis of the drug metabolising microsomal enzymes is enhanced by a number of commonly used drugs , insecticides and polycyclic hydrocarbons. This reduces the efficacy and increases the therapeutic dose of drugs metabolized by the microsomal enzymes.
- Inhibition : inhibition of the metabolism of one drug by another may lead to toxicity of the former. For example Allopurinol may inhibit metabolism of tolbutamide , methotrexate and probenecid and increase their toxicity.

(5) Interference with drug excretion :

- Excretion of weakly acidic drugs like sulphonamides , salicylates and barbiturates can be enhanced by making the urine alkaline.
- Probenecid inhibits the tubular secretion of penicillin , indomethacin and riboflavin thereby elevating their blood levels.
- Quinidine , verapamil and amiodarone can double the plasma digoxin concentration

(6) Receptor site interaction :

In this case , drugs acting on the same receptor site or at different active receptors may enhance or decrease the response . Example : tubocurarine and aminoglycoside antibiotics may accentuate the block at the neuromuscular junction ; marked CNS depression is caused by concurrent administration of morphine and barbiturates.

(7) Allopathic – Ayurvedic drug interactions :
Use of Allopathic and Ayurvedic drugs concomitantly has led to potential chances for interactions between the drugs of two systems. Few important examples follow :
- Guggulu is known to interact with hypolipidemics, anticoagulants, antihypertensives and thyroid medications.
- Concomitant use of castor oil reduces the efficacy of antiarrhythmic drugs, diuretics, fat-soluble vitamins and antihistamines.
- Yashtimadhu increases potassium loss and so prolonged use with thiazide and loop diuretics may be harmful.
- bleeding tendency after intake of
    - Phenprocoumon (a courmarin anticoagulant) along with ginger,
    - Warfarin (another coumarin anticoagulant) with Fenugreek, garlic, mango
- decrease in activity of Lithium (mood stabilizer) when consumed along with herbal diuretics like *Tribulus terrestris*, *Syzygium cuminii*.
- Loss of seizure control by Phenytoin (an anti epileptic) when combined with Ayurvedic herb *Shankapushpi.*

CHOOSE ALLOPATHY MAINLY FOR THE FOLLOWING :
1) All acute life threatening emergencies and many infections
2) Surgical issues like cataract , advanced arthritis (for joint replacement surgery) , cancers , many benign tumours , prostate enlargement , rectification of deformities and congenital anatomical abnormalities like cleft lip / cleft palate , nasal polyps etc.
3) Allergic rhinitis , vasomotor rhinitis
4) Chronic kidney failure with need for dialysis or renal transplant surgery
5) Bronchial asthma
6) Ophthalmic conditions like refractive errors , retinopathies
7) Hypothyroidism
8) Diabetes mellitus
9) Hypertension
10) Bleeding and clotting disorders
11) Inborn errors of metabolism
12) Diseases diagnosed by genetic studies for which there are no equivalents in other pathies

CONCLUDING REMARKS :

Allopathy is the undisputed pathy to be chosen for treatment of life threatening and other acute emergencies and diseases for which surgery is the definitive treatment (cataract , knee replacement surgeries etc). Advances in pathology and radiology make disease diagnosis mandatory before giving treatment and mankind owes a lot to these branches of modern medicine for revolutionizing medical practice. When it comes to predictability , reproducibility and promptness of clinical results Allopathy once again leads the way.

Advancements in modern surgical techniques are so highly impressive that for conditions like osteoarthritis of knee , cataract , benign superficial tumours like lipoma , cosmetic issues like gynaecomastia etc I would always recommend my patients to give top priority to surgical management. It drastically improves quality of life.

Because of unfair unwarranted media publicity side effects of modern medicines are exaggerated and in reality very few patients exhibit serious side effects of modern medicines. However , Allopathy falls short of tackling many chronic diseases which plague modern life and also has no solutions for peculiar troublesome clinical features for which treatment is available only in Homeopathy.

HOMEOPATHY

(Homeos : Similar ; Pathos : suffering)

INTRODUCTION TO HOMEOPATHY :

Homeopathy is a gentle but effective form of treatment which stimulates the natural ability of the organism to heal itself.

The word homoeopathy comes from the greek words "homeos" which means similar, and "pathos" which means disease. Homeopathy is a sophisticated method of individualizing small doses of medicines derived from plant , mineral and animal kingdom to initiate the healing response.

It was conceived in 1796 by the German physician Samuel Hahnemann who himself was a conventional medicine doctor. Samuel Hahnemann was a genius of unparalleled intellect way ahead of his times and hence rightly revered as Father Of Homeopathy.

History shows that Homeopathy has seen both good and bad days. Homeopathy achieved its greatest popularity in the 19th century. It was introduced to the United States in 1825 with the first homeopathic school opening in 1835. Throughout the 19th century, dozens of homeopathic institutions appeared in Europe and the United States. During this period, Homeopathy was able to appear relatively successful, as other forms of treatment could be harmful and ineffective. By the end of the century the practice began to wane, with the last exclusively homeopathic medical school in the US closing in 1920. In the 1970s, Homeopathy made a significant comeback, with sales of some homeopathic products increasing tenfold. The trend corresponded with the rise of the New Age movement, and may be in part due to a preference for "natural" products, and the longer consultation times homeopathic practitioners provided.

In the 21st century a series of meta-analyses have shown that the therapeutic claims of Homeopathy lack scientific justification. As a result, national and international bodies have recommended the withdrawal of government funding for Homeopathy in healthcare. National bodies from Australia, the United Kingdom, Switzerland and France, as well as the European Academies' Science Advisory Council and the Russian Academy of Sciences have all concluded that Homeopathy is ineffective and hence stopped further funding for research into its efficacy. The National Health Service in England no longer provides funding for homeopathic remedies and asked the Department of Health to add homeopathic remedies to the list of forbidden prescription items. France is looking to remove funding by 2021 while Spain has also announced moves to ban Homeopathy and other pseudotherapies from health centers.

PRINCIPLES OF HOMEOPATHY :

Hippocrates, the 'Father of Modern Medicine', taught that diseases could be treated according to the principle of contraries (contraria contrariis curantur) or of similars (similia similibus curantur). These recommendations were followed by later medical schools . Currently, the principle of contraries is massively employed in conventional therapeutics.

Homeopathy is based on the principle of - Similia Similibus Curentur – or in simple words – Like Cures Like. Thus , illnesses are cured by remedies or medicines which produce the same set of symptoms or signs when given to healthy people in potentized form. (We shall see what is potentized form in a short while).

For example , sulphur in material as well as potentized form produces burning when given to healthy people. Hence , sulphur in potentized form will remove burning from a patient when it is part of an illness.

Similarly , coffee heightens alertness and reduces sleep atleast initially in healthy people. Hence , coffee in potentized form will induce sleep in an insomniac when repeated thoughts prevent sleep.

HOMEOPATHY HAS A DRASTICALLY DIFFERENT APPROACH AS COMPARED TO ALLOPATHY AND AYURVEDA:

Let me explain this with the help of an example.

Suppose a patient comes with complaints of gradually increasing weight in spite of low appetite , dryness of skin , intolerance to cold, swelling in central portion of neck anteriorly , low heart rate , reduced muscle reflexes etc. The Allopathic doctor suspects hypothyroidism and this ***disease diagnosis*** gets confirmed by thyroid function testing. Levothyroxine is started and repeated thyroid function tests at 3 monthly intervals show improvement in values. Thus what has been approach to diagnosis ? Careful medical history , clinical examination , formulation of a diagnosis in mind and its confirmation by appropriate lab tests.

If the same patient would have presented to Ayurvedic doctor , same thought process would have been followed , hypothyroidism would have been suspected and same lab tests would have been ordered. Thus , even Ayurvedic doctor would first want to have a ***disease***

<u>*diagnosis*</u> before starting treatment. The exact word used to indicate diagnosis would obviously be different because language is totally different. While selecting medicine Ayurvedic doctor would have considered body type constitution of patient and selected appropriate medicine.

Coming to Homeopathy , matters become much more difficult or challenging. Homeopath has to follow the same procedure as Allopathic and Ayurvedic doctor to arrive at disease diagnosis. **But he needs 2 more things for success of treatment. A person diagnosis and miasmatic interpretation.** Disease diagnosis will tell the homeopath what disease patient is having. Person diagnosis will tell the homeopath what sort of a person has that disease. Final remedy selection would depend on 3 things : disease diagnosis , person diagnosis and miasmatic interpretation. Thus , let us say that the above patient sweats a lot on face and occiput , craves eggs , is intolerant of milk , experiences coldness of feet and hands. None of these features have anything to do with disease diagnosis. They are characteristic attributes of the patient and help remedy selection – calcarea carb in above case. This calcarea carb will ultimately bring down TSH and elevate the low thyroid hormones just the way levothyroxine does. Thus end result would be the same , approach being totally different.

If one silently ponders upon this piece of information , it will be noted that such peculiarities could be innumerable and likely to be totally overlooked by patient. **Hope doctors of other pathies understand now why practice of Homeopathy is so very difficult and challenging. Now one would start understanding why Homeopathy fails and why it produces miraculous results when perfect remedy is obtained.**

Practice of Homeopathy is both science and art. It is science because its based on logic , experimentation and scientific scrutiny. Its an art because during actual practice homeopath has to apply his own artistic skills to derive crucial information from patient for medicine selection – something which simply cant be explained adequately in books. Its an art which needs to be mastered with practice , practice and more practice.
This is somewhat similar to classical Indian music. There could be 10 singers trained in classical Indian music but the enjoyment that listeners would get by listening to each of them could be different. Science of music is the same – its application is an art.

MEDICINE DEVELOPMENT AND REMEDY SELECTION IN HOMEOPATHY :

Medicines in Homeopathy may be derived **from plant kingdom , animal kingdom or even chemicals**. Something as ubiquitous as table salt , as harmless as wood , as deadly as poison ivy can be used as medicine in Homeopathy.

Unlike in Allopathy or Ayurveda where medicinal substances are used in material doses or crude form , in Homeopathy they are used in potentized form. ***Potentization involves 2 things – (1) successive dilution of crude medicinal substance in alcohol / water / lactose and (2) revelation of its hidden medicinal power by thumping the medicine bottle on a firm resilient surface.***

Such a "potentized" medicine in varying degrees of dilution is administered to healthy human volunteers for a considerable period of time. While it is being administered , changes that take place in the volunteer are carefully recorded. These changes may be in form of subjective symptoms or objective signs. Homeopathic pathogenetic trials (HPT) are experimental studies to investigate the effects of potentially toxic or pathogenic substances serially diluted and agitated according to the recommendations in homeopathic pharmacopoeias on volunteers in good and stable state of health. HPT seek to produce valid and useful information on objective and subjective changes (mental, general and local) homeopathic medicines might cause in apparently healthy human beings. HPT are an evidence of the scientific nature of Homeopathy since its inception. HPT are one of the pillars of Homeopathy and a significant source of the symptoms, particularly mental, needed for prescription of homeopathic medicines. **The very huge database of these observations of thousands of medicines compiled in a systematic manner is what forms the "MATERIA MEDICA".**

Now when a patient naturally suffers from a disease , the homeopath goes into depths of these symptoms and signs and then searches the MATERIA MEDICA for the medicine which covers maximum of these signs and symptoms. Since materia medica is like a jungle of knowledge in which the homeopath feels lost , "REPERTORY" was developed to play the role of sign posts stuck to trees in the jungle which point towards group of remedies. **A "REPERTORY " is a listing of symptoms and those medicines that have been found to cause and cure each symptom.** Final remedy selection from this group takes place by close study of the MATERIA MEDICA to zero in on the closest matching remedy. In this search for the perfect homeopathic remedy common symptoms have lesser value. **The "peculiar , queer , rare and strange (PQRS) clinical features" have maximum value as far as selection of true similimum is concerned.** Such a remedy given in correct potency and repeated properly has the ability to produce miraculous results in the patient in form of quick relief of his / her symptoms.

The real challenge in day to day homeopathic practice lies in elicitation of these PQRS because they are usually ignored – being considered to be irrelevant to disease process by the patients.

The other closely competing remedies which share many signs and symptoms of the patient but don't match perfectly are partial similimums. When administered they will definitely remove some health problems of the patient but may not cure completely and may produce accessory side effects if given long enough.

Lock and Key analogy to understand variations in efficacy of homeopathic remedies – Lets imagine that disease is a lock inside which good health is trapped. Homeopathic remedies are keys to unlock it and liberate good health from shackles of disease. Now coming to lock and key analogy. Suppose there are 3 keys – 3 different homeopathic remedies selected by 3 different homeopathic doctors. One of them is totally wrong key (no similimum) , second one is partially correct key (partial similimum) and third is perfect key (true similimum). Using the first key there are no hopes that patient will feel better even after giving adequate time since the key just wont go in. The second key may go in and lock may loosen partially (partial improvement in health) and yet not be unlocked completely. The third key will go in smoothly , turn the internal wheels quickly and spring the lock open (complete improvement in health).

PROTOCOLS OF MEDICINE ADMINISTRATION IN HOMEOPATHY :

The principle and practice of Homeopathy has been detailed by its founder DR. Samuel Hahnemann in Organon. There are 6 editions of this book with each successive edition containing newer and newer insights into Homeopathy representing the cumulative experience of the master of Homeopathy.

As per the principles laid down In Organon in form of paragraphs or aphorisms, **only single dose of correctly selected homeopathic remedy should be administered followed by wait and watch policy.** This single dose supposedly provides a gentle nudge to the curative potential of dormant vital force awakening it back into action. Although at times this is followed in clinical practice , majority of the times homeopathic physicians advice the patient to take dose of medicine 3 times a day , 2 times a day , once a day , once a week etc depending on potency of medicine and response produced in patient.

Mother waking daughter analogy to help remember principles behind dose repetition of homeopathic remedies :

In order to remember the principles which govern frequency of repetition of homeopathic remedies let us take help of "mother waking daughter" analogy. Imagine a mother (homeopathic remedy) trying to wake up her fiery adolescent daughter (vital force which sets the healing ball rolling) snuggled up in bed in deep sleep.

Suppose the mother gives one wake up call and daughter wakes up and gets out of bed – would there be a need to give another wake up call ? No – isn't it? Similarly with just one dose if substantial improvement (more than 75%) occurs in health no need to give second dose immediately. Just wait and watch.

Suppose the mother gives one wake up call , daughter gets angry at being disturbed from her sleep , draws a pillow over face and refuses to get up. Any mother would know its wiser to wait for some more time before giving another wake up call – right ? Similarly after administering homeopathic remedy if symptoms worsen and homeopathic aggravation occurs its wiser to stop and observe , let the storm settle down and then decide further course of action.

Suppose the mother gives one wake up call , daughter just moves but goes back to sleep , mother gives another wake up call and daughter gets up and sits in bed and mother gives one more wake up call and daughter finally gets out of bed without any fuss. Similar to this when improvement in symptoms is noted to some extent say 10 – 40 % or so and with every dose further slight improvement occurs – that's the scenario in which to repeat.

Another occasion to repeat is when symptoms have improved , some time goes by and then they start worsening. That's the time to repeat. In the "mother waking daughter " analogy , after getting out of bed and moving about a bit if the daughter goes back to lie down in bed , obviously mother would have to once again give a wake up call.

Needless to say – this is just an analogy. In real life situation homeopathic or integrated medicine practice is far more complex. But anyway the above analogy at least helps to remember the approach to consider while deciding whether to repeat or not.

Hahnemann also suggested that only a single medicine should be used at any given time. This is no doubt followed by majority of homeopaths but others liberally use fixed dose combinations of multiple homeopathic medicines putting forth the argument that practically no one medicine covers all the important aspects of a patient's clinical history. Proponents and opponents of both methods – single medicine and FDCs galore , each trying to justify their own stance.

In my experience , both methods give results when used appropriately. Also what I have noted is - because patients often don't give PQRS symptoms - partial similimums get selected. They help partially but modify the totality and hence more than one medicines have to be used one after the other to ultimately cure the patient.

Hahnemann thought that the use of FDCs leads to over drugging of the patient and if several drugs are administered simultaneously , it is impossible to predict the synergistic effect. Selection of a single remedy based on the totality of symptoms requires deep study of the patient. However , selection of a single remedy doesn't mean that a single remedy will solve all problems of the patient during his life time. An acute or chronic case may require many remedies to cure.

Other points that patients on homeopathic treatment need to remember :
(1) Medicine globules should be placed either on or below tongue in a very clean odour free mouth. Presence of strong odours from food / medicines just consumed supposedly reduce the efficacy of homeopathic medicines. Hence patients are advised to keep a gap of 20 min to 30 minutes between consumption of meals and intake of homeopathic medicines. For the same reason if patient is simultaneously also taking Allopathic / Ayurvedic medicines its better to keep a gap of 1 hour minimum between various medicines.

(2) Patients are advised to avoid strong coffee , tea , smoking , alcohol , illicit drug use while on homeopathic treatment . Even something as harmless as handling camphor or strong essential oils may nullify medicinal benefits of homeopathic medicines. Hence one should not use or handle these strong smelled substances while on homeopathic treatment.

(3) Patient should take well balanced , nutritious diet , do regular exercise and get good refreshing sleep to speed up healing process.

(4) As soon as substantial improvement in overall health condition occurs , patient should start tapering off the medicines by reducing frequency of dosing. If worsening of symptoms is noted , next dose of same medicine should not be taken till remarkable improvement occurs and re occurrence of symptoms start.

(5) According to Homeopathy stalwart Dr. J. T . Kent patients respond to homeopathic treatment in 7 different ways. No response , direct simple amelioration , initial amelioration

followed by aggravation , similar aggravation , dissimilar aggravation , accessory symptoms , return of old symptoms (ROOS) are response patterns noted during homeopathic treatment. Years of experience are required before homeopath can correctly understand exactly what is happening to patient on treatment and suitably modify treatment in order to produce best results. Further , for the same reason continuous follow up and communication needs to take place between patient and homeopath after treatment is started. Give medicine and forget the matter – this never helps in Homeopathy. In fact , in some acute diseases homeopath may have to administer many homeopathic medicines one after the other in one single day to bring about complete cure. Patients need to remember this fact.

Good quality versus poor quality scooter accelerator analogy to help understand clinical response patterns noted on dose repetition of homeopathic remedies.
There are 2 kinds of accelerator response patterns shown by different scooters in Indian market. The accelerators of good quality scooters are such that increase in speed (acceleration) is proportionate to turning of accelerator handle. The accelerators of poor quality scooters are such that initially on raising accelerator increase in speed is disproportionately less whereas when accelerator cable is kept turned all of a sudden speed increases. Same thing happens in two clinical situations.
For reasons not clear , response shown by patients to administration of homeopathic remedies fall in above 2 patterns. Thus , in one pattern slight – moderate clinical improvement continues to occur as each dose is given. In second pattern , no improvement or at best slight clinical improvement occurs for few days and then there is a sudden improvement. An internationally famous homeopath with highly successful practice has openly told that he tells his patient to wait for 2 months before expecting to see response to treatment of chronic health problems.

UNDER WHAT CIRCUMSTANCES DO PATIENTS PREFER HOMEOPATHY AS PRIMARY MODE OF TAKING TREATMENT:
It's has always been a common experience of homeopaths that patients come to them at a very late stage of disease , often after unsuccessful Allopathic or Ayurvedic or other forms of treatment. However , of late this has changed and especially for day to day minor health complaints patients do prefer to take Homeopathy as treatment of first choice.

This change in attitude of some patients could be attributed to following reasons :
(1) Previous positive experience of Homeopathy

(2) Personal preference or family tradition

(3) Prefer Homeopathy due to its low cost

(4) Have experienced side effects of medicines of other pathies and would like to try Homeopathy because of its reputation of having no side effects.

(5) Traditional beliefs on immateriality or holism

(6) Awareness of the ineffectiveness of antibiotics for viral diseases and

(7) Mistrust of conventional medicine

I have mentioned before that there are some peculiar health complaints reported by patients which seem to defy logic and cant be explained by known facts in anatomy , physiology , pathology or other basic sciences. Such peculiar , queer , rare , strange (PQRS) features find solution only in Homeopathyc and following are just few examples :

(1) Cough with severe pain in distal parts (soles , palms , head etc) during coughing

(2) Innumerable delusions , illusions , body image distortions

(3) Tearing of eyes during urination or tearing of eyes on eating even less spicy food or tearing of eyes on exposure to dry cold air

(4) Blurring of vision during fever

(5) Face filled with sweat due to perspiration during eating always (not only during summer but every time)

(6) Ineffectual calls to move bowels during menses with experience of lower abdominal pain due to menstrual colic

(7) Bleeding from nose in a woman just before onset of menses or in lieu of menstrual flow

(8) Feeling of razor blades scratching throat during hawking

(9) Feeling of stone in pit of stomach or thread on tongue in it's actual absence

GREATEST OBJECTIONS TO HOMEOPATHY BY NON BELIEVERS :

(1) Homeopathy is a pseudo science and whatever few results are seen can be attributed only to the placebo effect.

The placebo effect is defined as a phenomenon in which some people experience benefit from a treatment because of positive expectations from it and not because of inherent merit of the treatment modality. After 24 years of studying Homeopathy I can definitely say that this defamatory statement is not true. Although prolonged interview by a kind , soft natured doctor showing sincere concern about patients health issues does have a placebo effect to some extent , definite changes in laboratory parameters of disease entities are hardcore evidence that Homeopathy does work beyond placebo effect. In fact , attempts to test effects of homeopathic medicines in modern laboratories by modern medicine doctors have shown changes even at gene expression level after giving homeopathic medicines.

Further , Homeopathy has shown to benefit unconscious , semi conscious patients , infants, animals like dogs , cats and even plants. In all these categories of subjects placebo effect is just not relevant. Disappearance of visible structural problems like warts , healing of ulcers which previously were not healing are sure shot evidences that Homeopathy acts beyond placebo effect.

(2) All relevant scientific knowledge about physics, chemistry, biochemistry and biology gained since the mid-19th century contradicts Homeopathy.

To some extent this objection is understandable because in spite of great efforts it has not been possible to show how homeopathic medicines produce beneficial effects in a vast majority of such occurrences. *" The fundamental implausibility of Homeopathy as well as a lack of demonstrable effectiveness has led to it being characterized within the scientific and medical communities as quackery and fraud "*:- I personally believe this statement is more out of ignorance about merits of Homeopathy rather than unbiased judgement.

Recently, demonstration that homeopathic medicines might modify cell functions through epigenetic mechanisms (DNA methylation and demethylation) has paved the road for a fully new field of research.

(3) There is no research in Homeopathy :

The skeptics of Homeopathy say that there is no research in Homeopathy. They probably do so because of lack of knowledge of research studies being done to elucidate mechanisms of Homeopathy or because such statements are common on internet and also made in few peer reviewed articles. The truth is that there are many studies on Homeopathy published in highly respected medical and scientific journals including THE LANCET , BMJ , PEDIATRICS , PEDIATRICS INFECTIOUS DISEASE JOURNAL , CHEST and many others.

Many clinical researches conducted on homeopathic medicines that have been published in peer reviewed journals , have shown positive clinical results especially in treatment of respiratory allergies , influenza , fibromyalgia , rheumatoid arthritis , childhood diarrhoea , recovery post abdominal surgery , attention deficit disorder and shown promising reduction in side effects of conventional cancer treatment.

In 2017 2 articles were published in journal "Cytokine" regarding research done to find out how homeopathic medicines act. In the first article it was reported that treatment of cutaneous Leishmaniasis patients with Antimonium crudum 30C might result in improvement of inflammatory lesions, but not in the elimination of infection. Antim crud was shown to interrupt monocyte migration to the primary lesion and hence when combined with parasiticidal medicines showed a synergistic effect.

In the second article it was shown that when Cantharis 6C was given to mice in which experimentally cystitis was induced by uropathogenic E coli , Cantharis induced changes in the distribution of the various leukocyte subtypes along the urinary tract mucosa. The bladder mucosa exhibited predominance of B cells compared to all other cell subtypes, while the pelvic mucosa exhibited greater concentration of T lymphocytes and macrophages. High concentration of B lymphocytes in the bladder implies greater local IgA production which facilitates the control of infection in the lower urinary tract. Thus , although homeopathic Cantharis did not have an antibiotic' effect it facilitated the host's adjustment to pathogens. When given along with antibiotics it is sure to have a synergistic effect.

 Dr. Khuda Buksh AR who has more than 100 articles in homeopathic research to his credit has shown that homeopathic potentized remedies act primarily through modulation of gene expression and has more than just a placebo effect.

A major research done in Brazil by Leoni Bonamin and team also demonstrated the preventive effects of homeopathic medicine prepared from the influenza virus.

In a double blind clinical trial employing Oscillococcinum 200C versus placebo in 487 patients diagnosed clinically to have influenza by 149 British general practitioners , the number whose symptoms subsided in 48 hours were twice in Oscillococcinum group compared to those in placebo group. Homeopaths who reviewed this study published In Lancet felt that results would have been much better if individualization would have been done for each patient receiving homeopathic medicine.

British Medical Journal published a double blind cross over clinical trial comparing use of Rhus Tox to placebo in patients of fibromyalgia (having symptoms for which Rhus Tox is indicated). Rhus Tox showed supremacy to placebo in statistically significant manner in reducing symptoms of fibromyalgia.

French researchers showed that potentized doses of Apis mellifica (crushed bee) and histamine has a statistically significant effect on reducing release of allergy causing chemicals from basophils.

(4) Homeopathy fails to deliver in many instances.

This objection , according to me is not fair. Failure to relieve patient of his health problems has been noted even when Allopathy and Ayurveda have been used. Does that mean they are pseudo sciences ? Medicine is a highly complex science and not a 100% science like mathematics. Failure of any remedy to act may be related even to factors such as poor quality of manufacturing of the medicine , poor patient compliance (taking few doses and skipping some) , wrong storage , inadvertent loss of effect due to exposure to strong chemicals , fumes , failure to wait for sufficient time for medicine to act. Wrong medicine selection could as well be because of factors beyond control of doctor such as inadequate or false history , wrong lab reports (either actual lab error or due to pre / post analytical factors) etc. *I am not saying this just to support a weak point. There have been so many instances in which even internationally famed stalwart homeopaths were unable to select correct homeopathic medicine with the result that patient could not be benefited. This was because of failure on part of patient to tell an important aspect helpful for medicine selection and when this important missing link came to surface and was used for medicine selection the same patient was totally cured of his disease.*

Homeopathy , of course cannot cure everything or everybody but it does offer the real possibility of cure for various deep seated acute , chronic and hereditary diseases.

WHY IS THERE SO MUCH RESISTANCE SHOWN BY SOME PATIENTS TO TAKE HOMEOPATHIC TREATMENT :

All sorts of patients exist in society. Some are more than willing to try various different modalities of treatment when they fall sick while others believe in sticking to time tested scientifically studied modalities of treatment only. Both of these approaches are relative with reference to time and experience – of self and of others - and there are various shades of attitude even amongst same class of patients.

In my experience , following are the reasons why some patients show extreme resistance to even thinking of taking homeopathic treatment when they fall sick.

(1) Previous bad experience where Homeopathy has not helped solve health issue and in fact health issue had worsened due to delay in starting Allopathic treatment

(2) Look down upon Homeopathy thinking it is poorly researched and appreciate the enormous data regarding scientific studies on various modalities of treatment especially in Allopathy

(3) Don't accept that a medicine which does not have even a single molecule of medicinal substance can produce any benefit to health

(4) Are aware that Homeopathy does require quite some time to show results especially in chronic complicated diseases and would rather prefer a quick solution to health problems.

ADVANTAGES OF HOMEOPATHY :
(1) It is safe, effective and cheap
(2) Chances of side effects are there but much less and many homeopathic medicines can be safely used in pregnant women and lactating mothers, infants and children and in the geriatric population
(3) In infections instead of killing microorganisms homeopathic remedies stimulate body's own "vital force " to fight against them. As such, no microbial resistance is known to develop against homeopathic medicines.
(4) The mode of administration of medicines is easy. There are no invasive methods and medicines are highly palatable, thereby enhancing their acceptability
(5) Lack of disease diagnosis is not a hindrance for initiating treatment with homeopathic medicines. Disease diagnosis is preferred but medicine diagnosis is mandatory.
(6) Homeopathic remedies are not addictive – once relief occurs, the patient can easily stop taking them
(7) Treatment is comparatively more cost-effective than other therapeutic systems.
(8) Drug sensitization , drug toxicity , drug resistance , allergies and anaphylactic shock do not occur while using homeopathic medicines in potentized form.
I would like to make few comments regarding this last point which I will cover in the first point under disadvantages of Homeopathy.

DISADVANTAGES / LIMITATIONS OF HOMEOPATHY :
(1) Homeopathic aggravations : After taking homeopathic medicine when symptoms -- for which treatment was being sought in the first place -- get aggravated its referred to as similar homeopathic aggravation. Most likely cause is too high a potency and / or too frequent repetition of homeopathic medicine.
Dissimilar homeopathic aggravations – akin to what is termed side effects in Allopathy / Ayurveda – also occur with use of homeopathic medicines. In fact life threatening killer homeopathic aggravations are known to occur when deep acting remedies are prescribed to patients with lowered vitality who have end stage organ diseases. So I feel that it is not true that homeopathic medicines don't show toxicity. Problem is with absence of research into why this happens and its documentation. Because such occurrences are not spoken of or

don't get documented every time they occur --- literature search fails to yield this information.

Thus , to summarize , it's a false boastful statement made by few homeopaths that side effects do not occur with Homeopathy. In practice they do occur. Their occurrence can be prevented by correct selection of remedy and administering it in correct potency and in apt dosing frequency.

(2) Tachyphylaxis or drug tolerance : Something similar to tachyphylaxis or drug tolerance does happen with use of homeopathic medicines also. Progressive decrease in reaction to same potency of correctly selected homeopathic remedy is known to occur. Hence its advised to give successive higher potencies to keep on curative effect when such observation is noted. Once again there is hardly any research into why this happens and no term is used for this phenomenon. To me , this is akin to phenomenon of tachyphylaxis or drug tolerance.

(3) Extremely difficult to select correct homeopathic medicine and high chances that information crucial to medicine selection may not get revealed in the first interaction between patient and homeopath thereby leading to second or third best remedy. I must admire the truthfulness of internationally famous stalwart homeopaths who have admitted to wrong medicine selection openly in their videos on youtube. Patient was not harmed because medicine selected was still quite close to patient totality.

As told elsewhere this difficulty is because of reliance in Homeopathy on those aspects of a person's totality which are usually unnoticed by the patient. One single PQRS symptom may point to the perfect remedy and when indeed its given to patient at times miraculous results are seen.

(4) Slow acting especially in chronic problems. For every one year of presence of a health problem it requires 1 to 3 months to eradicate the problem. On the other hand , if problem is of very recent onset Homeopathy can show results in seconds , even earlier than Allopathic medicines. Sadly, most patients come to homeopaths at very late stages of disease after having unsuccessfully tried treatment with all other pathies - and ironically expect immediate results from Homeopathy !!

(5) Unpredictability of results even when correct medicine gets selected. How to say that correct medicine has been selected ? Well … that's a question most difficult to answer because unlike Allopathy and Ayurveda where there are finite set of criteria on which medicine is selected , in Homeopathy the possibilities that result as an attempt is made to select right remedy (considering totality of clinical picture) are infinite. That is the reason why even in standard textbooks of Homeopathy there are sentences such as "when such and such remedy fails such and such remedy follows well and cures the patient". Further, well known expert homeopaths are known to give patients a set of medicines with the advice to take one of them and keep others as stand by. The stand by medicine is to be taken upon advice of homeopath after careful assessment of response to first prescription. Predictability of results is maximum in Allopathy , intermediate in Ayurveda and least in Homeopathy.

(6) Inability to work alone in some cases is another disadvantage :- In practice , for many patients homeopaths have to take help of Allopathy or Ayurveda to bring about substantial improvement in health. This occurs especially when advanced organ pathology has occurred and the PQRS features which help remedy selection are no longer present. Having said that , its equally true that Homeopathy has shown miraculous results in hopeless advanced cases rejected by and declared untreatable by Allopathy and Ayurveda.

(7) Mechanism of action of homeopathic medicines is not known : Whether or not one actually understands how homeopathic medicines work , this fact should not be be used to disprove efficacy of Homeopathy. Inaccurate explanations of gravity do not make it disappear and accurate explanations do not make it stronger. Likewise , inaccurate theories about how the homeopathic medicines work only discredit the explanation, not the method itself.

Thus , as readers would appreciate , I have given a very balanced and truthfull view of Homeopathy by dealing with both its advantages / pros and disadvantages / cons.

CHALLENGES IN FRONT OF HOMEOPATHY :
(1) Very poor funding or very poor encouragement given to Homeopathy by government
Conducting case control studies or randomized controlled trails requires huge money . It's the government's responsibility to fund this research. I am not saying its drug manufacturing company's responsibility because there are chances of biased reporting of research findings. If homeopaths want to furnish scientific evidence of efficacy of homeopathic medicines by pathology testing every time patient may not be ready to do so especially if tests are very costly and if repeated testing is required. In absence of funds and for fear of losing patient no attempt is made to document beneficial effects of homeopathic medicines.

(2) Inability to do quality control of homeopathic medicines. Since almost all homeopathic medicines (barring mother tinctures and very low potencies) don't have measurable medicine molecules and because all medicines look identical (liquid form or dry globules form) quality control to know if the watery liquid seen in medicine bottle is indeed homeopathic medicine is not possible. So , if manufacturing companies are indeed producing substandard medicines there is no way of proving or disproving that.

(3) Discredit brought by quacks and non medics practising Homeopathy : Selection of correct homeopathic medicine is a highly complex task requiring thorough clinical knowledge , knowledge of pathology , radiology , materia medica , organon and self experience gained over a life time. Dearth of competent homeopaths has made Homeopathy mutilated and emasculated. Homeopathy should not therefore be judged from results of many quacks that are prescribing Homeopathy and bringing discredit to this science.

(4) Difficulty in ascribing health benefit to homeopathic treatment. Let me explain this in form of an example. Let us say a patient suffering from severe acidity takes Allopathic medicine prescribed by Allopathic doctor and within minutes his complaints of acidity subside. Here its easy to give credit to Allopathic medicine because of clear cut association between medicine intake and health benefit noted. If acidity disappears with same speed after taking Homeopathy then its easy to give credit to it. However in very long standing health problems , it has been noted that the clinical benefit is slower in onset , very gentle and often noted when patient looks back in time after the homeopathic medicine has been taken for a few weeks – months. In the latter case patient may fail to give credit to homeopathic treatment.

CURRENT STATE OF HOMEOPATHY :
Acceptance of Homeopathy is going in 2 different directions in world today.
Increasingly more and more people world over are preferring to start treatment for their health issues with Homeopathy rather than as a last resort when nothing else helps. The growing popularity of Homeopathy has made it second most followed alternative therapy in the world. In many countries , the people seeking homeopathic care have crossed 30% which is likely to increase in coming century. This fast growing popularity has become a matter of concern to the mainstream medicine as it is posing a threat to their commercial gains.

Also many physicians from the other systems have started studying and practising Homeopathy today.

On the other hand , scientific bodies are rejecting Homeopathy. Many national and international bodies have recommended the withdrawal of government funding for Homeopathy in healthcare. National bodies from Australia, the United Kingdom, Switzerland and France, as well as the European Academies' Science Advisory Council and the Russian Academy of Sciences have all concluded that Homeopathy is ineffective and hence stopped further funding for research into its efficacy. The National Health Service in England no longer provides funding for homeopathic remedies and asked the Department of Health to add homeopathic remedies to the list of forbidden prescription items. France is looking to remove funding by 2021 while Spain has also announced moves to ban Homeopathy and other pseudotherapies from health centres.

PARADOXICAL PHARMACOLOGY – USE OF ALLOPATHIC MEDICINES THE HOMEOPATHIC WAY :

Along the past decade, pharmacologists suggested a therapeutic strategy named 'paradoxical pharmacology'. Similar to the one applied in Homeopathy for more than 2 centuries, it advocates the use of conventional drugs that cause a short-term exacerbation of disease to treat the very same disease in the long run.

In other words, using drugs which cause adverse events similar to the manifestations of disease to treat them homeopathically. This means employing the rebound effect (paradoxical reaction) with curative intention ;results are promising and indications countless.

Best example is of use of Ritalin (methylphenidate) an amphetamine like drug to treat hyperactivity in children. It is indeed ironic that physicians would consider giving an amphetamine like drug to children who are hyperactive. One would expect that such a drug would make the children even more hyperactive. But Ritalin has a noticeably opposite effect on such children. It calms them down and allows them to concentrate in studies or play. Allopaths refer to this action of Ritalin as "Paradoxical action "which in fact is just another name for homeopathic way of usage of modern medicines. The drug does not further relax children who are already calm , it only calms those who are hyperactive. Because Ritalin normally causes hyperactivity it can treat it effectively. However , Ritalin produces side effects such as nervousness , reduced appetite , weight loss , retarded growth and stomach aches , skin rashes , headaches and hallucinations.

CHOOSE HOMEOPATHY MAINLY FOR THE FOLLOWING :

1) Very early stage of common diseases where no diagnosis can be made and where clinical features are mild and vague

2) Patient gives PQRS (peculiar , queer , rare , strange) symptoms in history which cant be explained scientifically by known aspects of anatomy , physiology , pathology etc.

3) Where mental issues seem to be very much responsible for physical manifestation (psychosomatic disorders plus more)

4) Chronic conditions like allergies , asthma , migraine , acidity , skin problems , PCOD , sleep disorders , heel pain etc

5) Acute non serious conditions like common cold , cough , tonsillitis , pharyngitis , UTI , superficial bruises , cuts , wounds , diarrhoea etc.

A WORD ON BIOCHEMIC REMEDIES AND THEIR COMPARISON WITH HOMEOPATHY :

Biochemic remedies were first used in homeopathic practice by **Dr. Wilheim Schuessler** in the 19th century. They are formulated to support body's health and stimulate healing processes by regulating mineral levels in the body.

The 12 biochemic salts of Scheussler are :
(1) Cal fluor
(2) Cal Phos
(3) Cal Sulph
(4) Ferrum Phos
(5) Kali Mur
(6) Kali Phos
(7) Kali sulph
(8) Mag Phos
(9) Natrum Mur
(10) Natrum Phos
(11) Natrum Sulph
(12) Silicea

Although all biochemic remedies are also present as homeopathic remedies the potencies and mechanism of action are different. Biochemic remedies are available in potencies from 1X to 12X – most commonly used potencies being 3X , 6X and 12X. At this level of dilution material quantities of original substances can still be measured in samples of the medicine. Their action is said to be semi dynamic.

On the other hand homeopathic remedies are much more in number than biochemic remedies , are usually administered in potencies of C range – most commonly used potencies being 6C , 30C , 200C and 1M. Homeopathic remedies are said to act at dynamic level and dilutions are such that not a single molecule of original substance is present in any medicine.

Biochemic remedies are available only as white tablets unlike homeopathic medicines which are available as mother tinctures , liquid , sugar pills , creams , lotions , shampoos etc.

Usual starting dose for adults is 4 tablets 4 times per day with tapering off by reducing frequency as intensity of symptoms decrease. Tablets can be kept on tongue and sucked. Another way is to add few tablets in cup of water , dissolve and then take one tsp per hour etc

A WORD ON BACH FLOWER REMEDIES :

Dr. Edward Bach (a homeopath) created Bach Flower Remedies (BFR) in early 1900s. They are made out of watered down extracts from the flowers of wild plants.

Dr. Bach during his life time developed 38 flower remedies each addressing various personality or psychological issues. **In India , our own doctors : Dr. Rupa and Dr. Atul Shah have spent a lifetime researching , developing and clinically using effective flower remedies from Indian flowers.**

It's often said that there is no medicine for behaviour or inbuilt nature of a person. BFR and homeopathy does , in fact , have the power to change inbuilt nature or behaviour of a person – slowly but steadily and for a long long time.

The emotional issues which can be tackled using BFR are :

(1) Fear : of known or unknown

(2) Uncertainty

(3) Apathy to surroundings or society

(4) Loneliness

(5) Oversensitivity to influences and ideas

(6) Sadness or despair

(7) Cares for others at the expense of self

Names and uses of few BFR :

(1) Agrimony : for those who hide their worries from others under a cloak of cheerfulness and good humour.

(2) Heather : for the talkative self absorbed people who fear loneliness.

(3) Aspen : fear of unknown

(4) Mimulus : fear of the known

(5) Cerato : inability to trust ones own judgement , knowledge and intuition.

(6) Beech : for the perfectionist who tends to be intolerant of other peoples methods and experience.

(7) Centaury : For those who lack the will power to refuse the demands of others and so become willing slaves.

(8) Chestnut bud : for those who are slow to learn even from repeated mistakes or experiences.

(9) Gentian : Negative outlook , melancholy , discouraged when things go wrong or when there are difficulties.

Practical way to take Bach Flower Remedy :
You make a Bach Flower treatment bottle by adding 2 drops of each of the selected Bach Flower Remedies to a 30 ml/1 oz mixing bottle. You can combine up to 6 or 7 Remedies in a treatment bottle.
As preservative (optional) you can add 1 teaspoon brandy, apple cider vinegar or vegetable glycerin.
You then fill the bottle to the top with water and from this mixture you take 4 drops, 4 times a day until you feel better.

Homeopathy versus Bach Flower Remedy :
There's a lot of confusion between homeopathic remedies and the Bach system, but the two are very different. Homeopathic medicines can be re-potentized by further dilution – so the process of energizing them never really stops. Maybe that is why they are so delicate. With BFR the energizing process stops at the point that the mother tincture is finished. More dilution, succession etc. has no impact. The energy is fixed, which is maybe why Bach Remedies are so much less fragile than homeopathic remedies, and why we can take them in tea, coffee, food etc. in ways that would make a homeopath turn pale!

--- ≈≈≈≈≈ ◉ **Multi – Pathy Co – relation** ◉ ≈≈≈≈≈ ---
Integrating use of BFR into medical practice :
Since BFR are gentle , effective and without side effects they can be used to complement ongoing medical treatment with other pathies. This can be better understood by following example. Suppose there is a road traffic accident where fortunately there is no fatality but the victims are mentally shaken or in shock and are suffering from non fatal physical injuries. BFR Rescue remedy can be administered to them and will quickly help reduce the mental impact of the unexpected tragic event. Allopathic anti emetics can help reduce vomiting and injectable pain killers can substantially reduce pain. Allopathic vaccine like tetanus can help prevent development of tetanus in near future. Arnica / Bryonia / Rhus tox homeopathic medicines can help kick start healing process. Calendula cream can be applied locally to superficial cuts or abrasions. Ayurvedic pradhaman nasya can help revive an unconscious patient.

<u>Bach Flower Remedies and Pregnancy :-</u>
Bach Flower Remedies are extremely helpful during pregnancy, when the expecting mother goes through a wide range of emotions. The Bach Flower Remedies restore peace of mind

when the mother feels fearful, tired, overwhelmed and impatient and other emotions related to pregnancy. Rescue Remedy and Walnut are very useful during labor. All medication taken during pregnancy should be only after treating doctor's consultation and permission.

Bach Flower Remedies and Children :-

Children respond very well to the Bach Flower Remedies. The Bach Flower Remedies are extremely helpful for all childhood emotions such as: shyness, tantrums, fear, nightmares and low self-esteem. The Bach Flower Remedies help children reach a balance within themselves so that their reactions to situations are more controlled and less erratic.

Bach Flower Remedies for pets :-

Pets also have emotions and the Bach Flower Remedies are very helpful to aid pets overcome difficult times. The Bach Flower Remedies have been very successful in calming hyperactive dogs, fearful cats, trips to the vet, moving, fear of thunder, newly arrived puppies or kittens and many other pet emotions. If indeed this fact is repeatedly and reproducibly noted then it's a very strong argument against anyone who says that BFR act via placebo effect.

Can BFR be overdosed ?

It is impossible to overdose with the Bach Flower Remedies, they are 100% natural and safe. You can drink a whole bottle of Remedies and not "overdose.". However, if you think that "more is better" you are wrong. The Bach Flower Remedies work best over a period of time, taken from the treatment or stock bottle at least 4 times a day.

SIMILARITIES BETWEEN THE 3 PATHIES :

(1) Medicines used in all 3 pathies are sourced from plants , minerals and animals :

It's a misconception that all Allopathic medicines are harmful chemicals synthesized in laboratory and hence produce more side effects in human body. This is just not true.

Examples of some Allopathic medicines derived from plant sources are :

- Theophylline (a bronchodilator) is derived from black tea and green coffee beans
- Morphine , codeine , opium used for pain relief and illegal recreation are derived from the Opium Poppy (Papaver somniferum).
- Caffeine : used to treat fatigue and migraines is found in coffee beans, tea leaves etc
- Aspirin : contains salicylic acid which is derived from willow bark
- Digitalis : used to treat heart failure is derived from foxglove (digitalis purpurea)
- Quinine – an anti malarial drug is derived from bark of cinchona tree
- Paclitaxel (Taxol) a chemotherapeutic agent used in oncology is derived from bark of Yew tree
- Vincristine and vinblastine are alkaloids taken from the Madagascar periwinkle plant . Both are intravenous chemotherapeutic agents used for cancers like Hodgkin's disease and neuroblastoma.

Everything that is herbal is not necessarily safe. Nicotine and marijuana are herbal too. At the same time everything made in labs is not dangerous or artificial. In fact a lot of herbal products are made synthetically in factories or are cleaned , packaged or purified in factories , making then just as artificial.

Another misconception in this regards is that all Ayurvedic medicines are derived from plants and never from any animals. Again this is not true. On the basis of their origin, Ayurvedic medicines are also classified into three groups:

(1) kastha ausadhis (herbal preparations)

(2) rasa ausadhis (metallic preparations [e.g., bhasmas, sindoora])

(3) jangama ausadhis (animal preparation — prepared from animal products).

In India, nearly 15–20 percent of Ayurvedic medicines are derived from animal-derived substances. There are references to nearly 380 types of animal substances in Charaka

Samhita The Hindu religion has used five products (milk, urine, dung, curd and ghee) of the cow for purification since ancient times.

Noteworthy is the observation that mostly animal byproducts are used in traditional health care systems without any loss to animal.

Examples of some Ayurvedic medicines derived from animal sources are :
- Cow's urine used as a detoxifier , against cancer , in some viral diseases etc
- Goat's milk has been found to have similar healing properties to olive oil and regular consumption is recommended as a home remedy for anaemia, magnesium deficiency, eczema and acne. It also boosts the regeneration of haemoglobin and can be beneficial for those with osteoporosis.
- Legs of Indian peafowl are used to treat ear infection
- Dung of asiatic wild ass is used to treat jaundice
- Ash derived from the hard upper shell of Indian tent turtle is used in cough and lung diseases (asthma , TB etc)

Not only animals sources but animals themselves have been used for therapeutic purposes in Ayurveda. Use of leech (blood sucking animal) for some skin diseases is well known.

Even Homeopathy has some plant derived medicines such as :
- Andrographis paniculata (Kalmegh) used as mother tincture in Homeopathy as well as an Ayurvedic medicine
- Azadirachata indica (Neem) used as potentized medicine in Homeopathy and is of course a very well known Ayurvedic medicine
- Boerhaavia Diffusa (Punarnava) used as mother tincture in Homeopathy as well as an Ayurvedic medicine for edema.
- Brahmi is used as mother tincture in Homeopathy as well as an Ayurvedic medicine for impaired memory (as a nootropic agent)
- Coleus aromaticus (Pashanbhed) used as mother tincture or potentized medicine in Homeopathy and as Ayurvedic medicine for urinary tract stones.
- Gymnema Sylvester used against diabetes in both Homeopathy and Ayurveda
- Janosia asoka or Ashoka tree – used as mother tincture , 2x , 3x in Homeopathy and is a well known cardiac tonic in Ayurvedic medicine.

and some animal derived medicines such as :
- Badiaga : from skeleton of fresh water sponge
- Corallium rubrum : from skeleton of red coral
- Sepia : from ink of cuttlefish
- Asteria rubens : from star fish (whole animal)
- Aranea diadema : from cross spider (whole animal)
- Tarentula cubens : from Cuban spider (whole animal)
- Tarentula Hispania : from Spanish spider (whole animal)
- Apis mellifica : from honey bee (whole animal)
- Blatta americana : from American cockroach (whole animal)
- Blatta orientalis : from Indian cockroach (whole animal)
- Formica rufa : from ant (whole animal)

Its amply clear from above examples that medicines used in all 3 pathies are derived from plants and animals in addition to other sources such as minerals.

Homeopathic medicines derived from animal origin should be acceptable even to strictest of vegetarian patients because after the 12 C dilution the homeopathic medicine will not have even a single molecule of the original animal source from which medicine is made. Thus logically consumption of homeopathic medicines made from animal sources should not offend religious sentiments of even hardcore vegetarians (so long as dilution is more than 12 C).

At times source of medicine is plant or animal but the final medicine derived from it is lab synthesized – being an isolated substance from source in natural form.

(2) Same medicine may be used by more than one pathy for the same purpose :
- Best example of this is use of Sarpagandha in Ayurveda , reserpine alkaloid derived from Sarpagandha (Rauwolfia serpentina) in Allopathy and Reserpine mother tincture in Homeopathy for treatment of hypertension
- The seed powder of the leguminous plant, Mucuna pruriens has long been used in Ayurveda Indian medicine for treatment of Parkinsonism. Levodopa / carbidopa combination has been used in Allopathy for treatment of Parkinsonism. The link between the two is that seed powder of mucuna pruriens (kaunch bee) contains significant quantities of Levodopa.

- Belladonna (or Atropa Belladonna) is a plant from which two important alkaloids – atropine and scopolamine are derived. In Ayurveda , extracts of Belladonna are used for relieving pains and for decreasing mucous secretions in patients with cough and asthma. In Allopathy , atropine preparations are used as intestinal antispasmodic to control colicky pain , with morphine in treatment of biliary colic, in ophthalmology to produce mydriasis and cycloplegia , to reduce respiratory secretions and thereby prevent laryngospasm during anaesthesia , in organophosphorus poisoning , in Parkinsonism etc. Belladonna is a very commonly used medicine in Homeopathy especially for acute conditions presenting with heat , redness , throbbing and burning.

- Aesculus hippocastanum or horse chestnut is a tree . Horse chestnut seed extracts are most commonly taken by mouth in Ayurveda to treat varicose veins and other circulatory problems that can cause the legs to swell. Mother tincture and potentized versions of Aesuclus hippocastanum are used even in Homeopathy for varicose veins and piles.

- Softgels and tablets derived from garlic (allium sativum) are used in Ayurveda as supplements for heart and high bp patients because of vasodilatory and blood thinning properties of garlic and because of its salutary effects of lipid profile. Similarly mother tincture of allium sativum is used in Homeopathy to reduce blood pressure. In potentized form garlic is used in Homeopathy for pain in hip , pain in psoas and iliac muscles.

- Gold has been used as medicine in all 3 pathies. In Allopathy , gold has been used with variable success rate in treatment of rheumatoid arthritis , as injection of microscopic gold pellets in the treatment of prostate cancer and in some immunosuppresants as gold nanoparticles. In Ayurveda gold containing FDCs like Sutshekhar Ras Gold is used to lower body temperature and relax mind , Saraswatarishta with gold is used for depression and for improvement of cognitive functions , Swarna Bhasma mixture for dry cough , Vasant Malti Ras (Gold) along with other medicines to treat recurrent tonsillitis , Mahayograj guggul gold for rheumatoid arthritis. In Homeopathy potentized versions of aurum metallicum (gold metal) have been used for various indications such as endogenous depression , extreme photophobia , high blood pressure with violent headache etc.

- Marigold flower preparations are used in Ayurveda for psoriasis. In Homeopathy aqueous calendula (derived from calendula Officinalis or marigold) is used for all wounds.

- Saffron (Crocus Sativa) is used in Ayurveda in skin care preparations and in potentized form in Homeopathy for black and stringy hemorrhages.

(3) Side effects may be produced by consumption of medicines of all 3 pathies :

When I began in depth study of Ayurveda and Homeopathy in addition to Allopathy (of which I had formal official training for 8 and ½ years) I was made to believe by media and society that only Allopathic medicines have side effects and usage of Ayurvedic and homeopathic medicines is never associated with side effects. Now – after many years of practical working experience with use of medicines of all 3 pathies - I can confidently say that side effects may be produced by consumption of medicines of all 3 pathies. Happily though I would like to point out that incidence of side effects is much less when medicines are used correctly – Allopathic , Ayurvedic or homeopathic.

Although anecdotal or hearsay evidence suggests that side effects are relatively more when Allopathic medicines are used (maximum 10% of all clinical instances of their consumption) its difficult to be sure of side effects by Ayurvedic and homeopathic fraternities in the absence of in depth scientific studies and unbiased reporting.

Causes of adverse drug reactions told in Ayurveda can be grouped under follow headings :

1. Drug interaction (Viruddadravyaprayoga)

2. Iatrogenic (Vaidhyakruti)

3. Over dose (Atimatradravyaprayoga)

4. Administration of unwholesome drugs (Ahitatamadravyas)

5. Administration of medicine in diverse pathological stages (Avastanusaradravyaprayoga)

6. Therapeutic procedural complications (Panchakarmavyapad)

7. Improper use of Rasaushadi (Medicines of mineral origin)

Examples of side effects produced by Ayurvedic medicines :

- Lead toxicity by consumption of Ayurvedic bhasma of poor quality or their usage for a long time. Elevated lead levels , presence of lead lines on gums and basophilic stippling noted in RBCs on peripheral smear are evidences to support this toxicity.
- Arsenic toxicity by consumption of Ayurvedic bhasma of poor quality or their usage for long time. Elevated blood arsenic levels and presence of Mee's lines in nails are evidences to support this toxicity.
- Hypoglycemia is a known side effect of many anti diabetic Ayurvedic herbs

- Constipation is a known side effect of kutajarishtha or other preparations where kutaja is used or if kutaja is used in high doses for longer periods of time
- Side effects of consuming Bacopa monnieri may include dry mouth, thirst, nausea, indigestion, increased regularity of bowel movements, drowsiness, fatigue, or palpitations. Bacopa might slow down the heartbeat. This could be a problem in people who already have a slow heart rate.
- Women who are currently suffering from heavy menses should avoid Jatamansi because it will increase menstrual blood loss.
- Consumption of the non deglycyrrhinated form of Licorice or mulethi in high doses has an aldosterone like effect leading to high blood pressure.
- In a few women with high estrogen levels, Shatavari raises estrogen levels further leading to water logging and breast tenderness.
- Triphala may cause loose stools and abdominal pains / cramps
- Trikatu may lead to heartburn in patients predisposed to acidity because of black pepper / long pepper content.
- High dosage and unwise use of Akarkara can lead to excess mouth salivation and even mouth ulceration
- The most common side effect of vacha (acorus calamus or sweet flag) is headache
- Unwise use of sarpagandha can cause nasal stuffiness and dryness of mouth
- Some people can experience the following side effects with Kanakasava: Headache , Nausea , vomiting and restlessness
- Long-term use of aloe vera may result in loss of potassium and other electrolytes.
- The common side effect of Khadirarishta is burning sensation or heartburn. It generally occurs when Khadirarishta is taken without mixing water.
- Kumaryasav when taken in wrong doses can exacerbate bleeding of bleeding piles
- Anu Thailam causes mild irritation in the nose, throat and mouth. You can also feel nasal congestion due to excess secretions immediately after using it.
- Unsupervised direct use of mukta wati can lead to nasal congestion , dry mouth and light headedness
- Pitta symptoms (heartburn , hyperacidity etc) may worsen when Ayaskriti is taken by people with aggravated Pitta conditions
- Intolerance to Saraswatarishtha may lead to indigestion , acid reflux , constipation , vomiting or nausea , high blood pressure , low blood sugar level (patient may complain of increased irritability) and palpitation

- Lakshadi guggul can cause following side effects if ingested in heavy dosages (more than 6 grams per day) : Stomach upset , headache. Allergic reaction to any of its ingredient can result in itching, hives and skin rashes.
- The excess use of Mrit Sanjeevani Sura can result in following side effects : loose stools drowsiness , upset stomach , headaches , mild nausea
- The long-term use or high dosage of Sphatika Bhasma can cause the following side effects : mouth dryness , gastritis , ulcers (it can occur with high dosage),nausea and vomiting (it can occur with high dosage and if Bhasma is raw and not well-processed.)
- The excess dosage or wrong administration of Tamra bhasma can result in severe side effects including :- nose bleed , high blood pressure , anal fissure , mouth ulcer , vertigo , nausea , vomiting , diarrhea and bleeding disorders
- Kanchanar guggulu may produce following side effects in sensitive people : stomach upset or mild gastric irritation , itching or skin rash , loose stools , hiccups etc
- Side effects of tagara may include : hypotension, light headedness, hiccup, nausea, and vomiting.
- Disorders like impotency, dryness of mouth, refractive error, lean, fainting and diarrhoea are result of over usage of *Commiphora mukul,* curd, *Piper longum,* salt, alkalis and administration of single flavoured items (*Ekarasasevana*)
- Excess intake of drugs with similar action on human body : like administration of paste of *Operculina turpethum* along with *Ichhabhedi ras* (Herbal formulation) causes drastic purgation

With so many examples given its adequately clear that Ayurvedic medicines – even herbal ones – can be associated with unwanted side effects. However if used under guidance of an expert Ayurvedic doctor and if due precautions are followed incidence of side effects can be kept very low.

Understanding concept of side effects and noting their presence in Homeopathy is highly complex . May be that is the reason why - even when side effects are shown by patients - they are not labelled as such by homeopaths and patients alike. The 2 common reasons responsible for side effects during homeopathic treatment are :
(1) improper potency of medicine
(2) improper dosage or frequency of repetition of medicine.

Side effects due to homeopathic medicines are termed as homeopathic aggravation which can be of 2 types :

(1) Similar homeopathic aggravation in which symptoms for which medicine is being given increase for a short duration of time (few minutes to few hours) and then subside.

Although not needed and obviously not desired for successful homeopathic treatment , many homeopaths are happy to note similar homeopathic aggravation because it is a sure-shot indication that remedy is working and will totally remove symptoms of the patient. Wise homeopaths pre warn the patients about such an aggravation.

(2) Dissimilar homeopathic aggravation is closest to what is regarded as side effects in Allopathy and Ayurveda. Here patient may report new symptoms developing. It requires considerable clinical knowledge of natural course of disease being treated in addition to knowledge of proving symptoms of medicines and sensitivity profile of patient in order to correctly infer what is going wrong in the patient. There is a concept in Homeopathy called proving of medicine. When repeated doses of specific dilutions of one homeopathic medicine is given to healthy volunteers - after some doses - volunteers start exhibiting some symptoms. This is known as drug proving. These symptoms are carefully noted to decide which homeopathic medicine can be therapeutically used to treat which symptoms of the patient. Some unfortunate hypersensitive patients start proving homeopathic medicines given to them to help reduce their suffering. Such patients are very difficult – almost impossible to treat by Homeopathy.

The difference between side effects of lab synthesized chemicals used as drugs and potentized homeopathic medicines is that they are usually minor and do not harm , poison or create addiction. They just indicate that the remedy has been given in too large a dose , too often , or in unsuitable potency. Once the remedy is stopped , they disappear. Some homeopaths believe that they are credited with having a strengthening effect on the person's vitality.

Another deadly side effect noted with administration of wrong homeopathic medicine at a wrong time in wrong doses is known as "killer homeopathic aggravation". If a deep acting homeopathic remedy is given to chronic complicated case (with various layers of disease processes superimposed one on the other) without prior preparation of the case by administration of a superficially acting related remedy , killer homeopathic aggravation endangering life of patient can develop. Such homeopathic aggravation may be seen with use of Sulphur , Arsenic or Lachesis – but is fortunately rare.

Its obvious from the above discussion that even so called safe therapeutic practices such as Ayurveda and Homeopathy can lead to harmful side effects in patients and hence its very very important that non medicos should not self treat even with Ayurvedic or homeopathic medicines. **There are high chances of endangering health if patients bypass doctors and take treatment by following advice given on google , youtube , directly from pharmacist or some inadequately qualified person.** I have written a very easy to understand article on this issue which has been published in this book as a bonus.

PARALELLS IN THEORY AND PRACTICE OF AYURVEDA AND HOMEOPATHY
Ayurveda and Homeopathy are the two widely used medical therapies in the world based on the constitutional approach and therapeutics. There are some parallels in concepts and practices of Ayurveda and Homeopathy.

We have seen before that Ayurveda promulgates the concept of 5 natural elements or Panchamahabhuta – namely Prithvi (Earth) , Apa (water) , Teja (fire) , Vayu (Air) and Akash (Ether). Based upon predominance of each of these natural elements in a person's body , Ayurveda believes there are 3 main body types : Pure Kapha , Pure Pitta and Pure Vata and their combinations : Kapha – Pitta , Vata – Pitta , Kapha Vata etc.
Certain homeopathic remedies selected as per constitution of patient show better actions in certain body types. Thus patient for whom Silicea is indicated is earthier , Nat mur is more with water element , Sulphur constitutes more fire element , Phosphorus is airy and Cannabis indica has a strong ether element.
Vata body types are known to be thin and homeopathic remedies Silicea , Phosphorus , Secale cor work better in thin individuals.
Kapha body types are known to be fat and round and homeopathic remedies Calcarea carb , Phytolacca are known to work better in fat individuals.
Pitta body types , although have an average body frame , they have fiery temperament and suffer form acidity. Lycopodium , Nux vomica medicines might work better in such individuals.

Regarding administration of medicines : - Ayurveda holds that the efficacy of medicine varies according to the time of intake of medicine. It is believed that efficacy of medicine taken in morning on empty stomach will be more effective. Medicines to induce sleep are obviously taken late in the evening.

Homeopathy also believes that medicines should be taken few hours before known times of aggravation of symptoms for which they are being prescribed. Thus Nux vomica is best given at bedtime while Sulphur is best given in the morning on empty stomach.

That Ayurvedic treatment involves some disease specific dietary restrictions or pathya is well known to patients. What many may not know is even Homeopathy advocates some restrictions such as restricted consumptions of coffee, tea, onion, garlic or emphasizes importance of avoiding strong smelled substances such as camphor , ammonia , glacial acetic acid , essential oils etc when consuming homeopathic medicines.

DIFFERENCES BETWEEN THE 3 PATHIES :

If one were to compare these 3 pathies with judiciary this is how they come out.

Allopathy is more like modern judiciary – passing judgements and trying to deliver justice while giving importance only to hard core facts – what can be submitted in the form of evidence.

Ayurveda is like the gram panchayat – passing judgement and trying to deliver justice by relying on age old traditional wisdom handed over by previous generations.

Homeopathy is much like a close family friend cum well wisher – passing judgements and trying to deliver justice by relying upon highly personalized knowledge of a person not accessible to any outside member.

Aim of all 3 is to give justice (improve health) but the approach is different.

Modern medicine (Allopathy) originated in Western world (America and Europe) , Ayurveda from India and Homeopathy from Germany. These 3 major treatment modalities differ in the following ways :

(A) RAPIDITY OF ONSET OF ACTION OF MEDICINES AND SPEED OF CURE / CONTROL OF SYMPTOMS:

After the patient takes a correct medicine in correct manner some time is required before symptoms start abating and health benefits are noted. In other words some time is required for onset of action of the medicines. This latency is because time is required for medicine to dissolve , be absorbed , get distributed to various tissues of body via blood and then exert its action by various mechanisms.

In my experience , Allopathy and Homeopathy compete closely with each other as far as rapidity of onset of results is concerned – at least in briefly existing acute diseases. Although beneficial effects of Allopathic medicines are more crystal clear , predictable and reliable , readers would be surprised to note that magical effects within short time have been noted by me not with Allopathy but with Homeopathy.

I will give you few examples :

(1) One patient had come to me on the way to office with very uneasy sensation in upper part of abdomen near the midline which both of us correctly attributed to entrapment of gas with difficulty in its expulsion by burping. This patient had no faith in Homeopathy and would always politely resist my suggestions at administering Homeopathy to him.

I knew of one homeopathic medicine which was definitely going to help him. Problem was that he would not take it. So I skillfully kept him busy talking , quickly made one dose , asked him to open his mouth and swiftly put 3 pills of that homeopathic medicine below his tongue. Within 2 seconds he was relieved of his uneasiness by induction of burping and release of the entrapped gas. He was surprised to note such rapid relief with Homeopathy.

(2) Another patient who was already feeling much better with my integrated treatment for Covid 19 came to me mid way during the treatment with extreme head pain in one round spot – a complaint pre – existing before he got Covid. The head pain was severe , as though blood was hitting that spot from inside. After enquiring into further details of his complaint I selected one medicine , gave him one dose , asked him to close his eyes and sit quietly for 10 minutes. After 10 minutes when he opened his eyes he told me that he felt much better , headache was much less. At home , the gushing of blood was experienced as pain 27 times per minute which reduced to 4 times per minute after that single dose. In next 5 minutes his headache disappeared completely.

(3) One patient suffering from cold , cough , fever , bodyache etc had already taken only allopathic treatment from a G.P before another patient brought him to me. He was not happy with the benefits of allopathic treatment and wanted me to give intravenous medication. After noting discrepancy between temperature and pulse rate and examining tongue etc I administered just one pill of one homeopathic medicine below his tongue. The patient was very dissatisfied with my approach and went away not so happy. After about 5 hours he called back to give feedback that the medicine had worked like magic and that he was bringing another patient for treatment !!

(4) One middle aged cricket lover was prohibited by Orthopedicians from playing cricket in view of his ankle and heel pain. His desire to play cricket was so much (after a gap of many years he was getting opportunity to participate in tournament) that he came to me to do something so that he could play. After thorough evaluation I gave him one biochemic and one homeopathic medicine. You will not believe – but in just one day his pain recued 95% . Although it recurred to a lesser extent later on it I adjusted the dosage and made changes in treatment such a way that he could play all matches of the tournament in near pain free manner. Within few more weeks time in spite of no rest his ankle / heel pain went away with continued homeopathic treatment.

Predictability of drug action and rapidity of effects places Allopathy at the forefront of treatment of acute life threatening emergencies and disease states requiring ICU admission. This is well known to everyone. What is not known by many - or known only by handful few - is that even Homeopathy can do wonders in similar situations. If so , then why isn't Homeopathy used frequently in acute emergencies ? Problem lies with the extreme difficulty of remedy selection , too much scarcity of skilled homeopaths with ability to tackle life threatening conditions and unpredictability of response (mainly because of inadequate experience of treating doctor).
Austrian doctors Dr. Michael Frass and Dr. Martin Bundner – both Allopathic physicians - have written a textbook titled : HOMEOPATHY IN INTENSIVE CARE AND EMERGENCY MEDICINE – in which they have described successful application of Homeopathy to intensive care and emergency department patients – at times with magical results.

What I have noted is – selection of correct homeopathic medicine from 4000 such – is an extremely difficult skillfull task requiring years of hardwork and experience. But when correct homeopathic medicine (true similimum) in correct potency is administered magical results are seen and can make difference between life and death for the patient.
In conditions such as status asthamaticus or pyogenic meningitis homeopathic medicines co - administered with modern medicines can reduce their requirement and improve end result.

When compared to Allopathy and Homeopathy health benefits from administration of Ayurvedic medicines are slow and do need much more time. However as alluded to before , now we know that Ayurveda has parasurgical techniques and some panchakarma protocols which produce amazing health benefits within seconds – minutes - hours when employed for emergency / acute onset health issues.

In the treatment of chronic complicated cases the thumb rule in Homeopathy is - for every one year of presence of a given symptom 1 to 3 months are required for its removal. So , if a patient has been suffering from say migraine for 3 years , any where from 3 to 9 months may be required for complete benefit. Benefits may start to manifest within few days but for complete recovery above mentioned time is required. Use of integrated medicine protocols may help shorten this time frame. The idea is to quickly bring about reduction in symptoms by starting with Allopathic and / or homeopathic medicines together with Ayurvedic medicines and try tapering them off (in order to prevent drug dependence) co inciding with onset of action of Ayurvedic medicines. This appears to be very simple in theory but in reality

, in practice this is a terribly complicated task testing the skill of the doctor. **This is one area where lot of research is still needed and government should give generous contribution to fundamental research in this new area so that new protocols for treatment of various diseases using integrated approach are designed.**

Another point that patient and practitioners should remember is that after beginning treatment , at times , no benefit may be seen while taking Ayurvedic and Homeopathic treatment for many days at a stretch and then all of a sudden symptoms start resolving. This occurs even during Allopathic treatment especially with usage of diuretics as monotherapy for hypertension and SSRIs for depression.

Lets move on to the next point of comparison.

(B) PREDICTABILITY OF RESPONSE TO TREATMENT :
Allopathic treatment leads the way in this matter. Beneficial effects and side effects after use of Allopathic medicines are much more predictable and well studied / well defined compared to Ayurvedic and homeopathic medicines.
Thus when Paracetamol is taken for bodyache induced by viral fever it will surely reduce the body ache. It matters not whether patient has faith in Allopathy - reduction in body ache will always be noted by the patient. Similarly when PPIs like Omeprazole , Esomoprazole , Pantoprazole are taken for acidity the symptoms of acidity surely reduce.
With use of other Allopathic medicines such as antibiotics the results are not always dependable because infection might be with bacterium resistant to the antibiotic which is being used. Same is true for medicines used in psoriasis or anti depressants where doctor needs to resort to little trial and error before zeroing on the perfect medicine.

Response to treatment is also quite predictable when Ayurveda is used – although less so as compared to Allopathy. Variations in composition of medicines by different manufacturers , lack of adherence to strict quality control procedures during manufacturing of medicines , less stringent pharmacovigilance , wrong applicability mismatched to kapha – vata – pitta status of the patient could be some of the reasons why this happens.

Unpredictability in response to treatment – with magical results when perfect homeopathic medicine is taken by same patient for same disease – is what I have noted as far as Homeopathy is concerned. Such unpredictable results are witnessed even when treatment is given by best of homeopaths – true homeopath stalwarts. May be that is the reason why there are sentences in homeopathic textbooks – when abc homeopathic remedy fails xyz remedy follows well and cures the disease. In fact its part of homeopathic therapeutics to administer intercurrent remedies (both nosodes and non nosodes) to remove what are termed as "miasmatic blocks" to expedite healing process. Miasmatic blocks refer to bodily conditions interfering with action of well selected homeopathic remedy producing discouraging clinical results.

Moving ahead with the next point of comparison……

(C) DEPENDANCE LIABILITY , REBOUND EFFECT AND ITS SIGNIFICANCE IN TREATMENT CONTINUATION , DISCONTINUATION AND SWITCHING FROM ONE PATHY TO THE OTHER :

Medicine dependence refers to the need to take medicine to keep on enjoying good health and to suffer from horrible side effects if medicine is stopped – either suddenly or after tapering it down slowly.

This is a highly complex but very important topic. I will try to explain it in simple language. Understanding this topic will help understand :

- Why Allopathic doctors usually advice patients to take some medicines life long
- Why sudden discontinuation of medicines (usually Allopathic ones) leads to reoccurrence of disease in more serious form
- What challenges a well intentioned doctor is likely to face when trying to reduce long term medicines of any patient
- Why one needs to always take treatment under proper medical guidance and not self treat , however minor the health issue may be
- Why there is need to integrate the 3 pathies and do intensive research to find out if this integration helps solve the problem of drug dependence

To understand drug dependence we need to know what is the meaning of PRIMARY and SECONDARY drug actions.

Lets try to understand these concepts with help of this example :-

Example 1 : use of antacids (Proton Pump Inhibitors like Omeprazole , esomoprazole , pantoprazole and others) in treatment of hyperacidity.

The "primary action" of antacids is to reduce HCL secretion in stomach by one way or the other. What happens because of this primary action ? Acid secretion reduces , hyperacidity abates and patient is relieved of symptoms such as retrosternal burning , waterbrash etc.

When antacids are indiscriminately taken for a long duration of time , stomach acidity remains lowered chronically (an abnormal state for human body). Human body tries its level best to bring it back to normal by increasing gastrin cell mass. These gastrin cells produce hormone gastrin which acts locally on adjacent acid producing cells thereby bringing about increased acid secretion. This is the "secondary action "or what can be termed "secondary reaction of body to primary action of the drug ".

What is the result of this secondary action → Over secretion of acid leading to rebound hyperacidity much more in severity than that present before treatment with PPIs was started.

Clinically how is this secondary action witnessed → Soon after completely stopping PPIs patient develops severe hyperacidity manifesting as intense retrosternal burning , waterbrash and pain in epigastrium. This occurs from the second week (half-life of PPI) to the normalization of the ECL cell mass (about 2 months), i.e., 2-3 months after treatment discontinuation.

What is done to get relief → drug dependence has occurred and one needs to restart the medicine and take it life long or taper it down very slowly.

Above is classical description of a "rebound effect ". **By definition, 'rebound effect' refers to production of increased negative symptoms when the effect of a drug has passed or the patient no longer responds to the drug.** If a drug produces a rebound effect, the condition it was used to treat may come back even stronger when the drug is discontinued or loses effectiveness. This is different from relapse of the original disease when original symptoms come back slowly and with same or reduced intensity.

How soon after stoppage of drug rebound effect is clinically noted depends on :

- half life of drug or its metabolite present in the body
- how intense was the therapy and how soon or rapidly the drug was discontinued.

Drug tapering rather than abrupt discontinuation minimizes the occurrence of the rebound effect.

Rebound effect might also occur along the course of treatment, in cases of therapeutic failure or development of tolerance, tachyphylaxis or receptor desensitization.

Let us see few more examples of drug dependence and rebound effect:

Example 2 : Drugs classically used for treatment of angina pectoris (β-blockers, calcium channel blockers, nitrates, and others) with beneficial effects through their primary action might trigger a paradoxical increase of the frequency and intensity of chest pain after discontinuation.

Example 3 : Drugs used for arterial hypertension (α-2 agonists, β-blockers, ACE inhibitors, MAO inhibitors, nitrates, sodium nitroprusside, hydralazine, and others) might produce rebound arterial hypertension once the primary biological effect ends.

Example 4 : Antiarrhythmic drugs (amiodarone, β-blockers, calcium channel blockers, disopyramide, lidocaine, mexiletine, moricizine etc) may trigger rebound exacerbation of arrhythmias if they are discontinued.

Example 5 : Antithrombotic drugs (argatroban, bezafibrate, heparin, salicylates, warfarin, clopidogrel etc) might promote thrombotic complications as result of the rebound effect.

Example 6 : Drugs such as statins which have vasculoprotective effects in addition to lipid lowering effects might cause rebound endothelial dysfunction, resulting in predisposition to paradoxical vascular accidents.

Example 7 : Sudden discontinuation of anxiolytics (barbiturates, benzodiazepines, carbamates etc), stimulants of the central nervous system (caffeine , , amphetamines, cocaine, methylphenidate etc), antidepressants (tricyclic antidepressants like amitryptiline , MAO inhibitors, selective serotonin reuptake inhibitors etc) or antipsychotics (clozapine, phenothiazines, haloperidol, pimozide etc) might cause rebound aggravation of the original condition after the end of their primary therapeutic effect.
Sudden withdrawal especially of the short acting anti depressants like Paroxetine and Venlaflaxine (having a very short half life) results in unbearable withdrawal symptoms comprising of brain zaps , nausea , vomiting , headache , tingling numbness , burning sensation in feet and hands , GI disturbances and mood swings. This forces patients to restart treatment with these anti depressants. Very gradual tapering also may not help much and patient is left with either no option but take these medicines life long or try to control symptoms of withdrawal syndrome using Ayurveda or Homeopathy.

Example 8 : Anti-inflammatory agents (steroids and NSAIDs) might trigger paradoxical increase of inflammation and rebound thrombosis when their use is discontinued . This occurs because of increase of COX-1 production and platelet activity (TXA2) to values higher than the ones before treatment. With this the odds for thromboembolic events (unstable angina (UA), acute myocardial infarction (AMI), stroke, and others) increase among susceptible individuals.

Example 9 : Analgesics (opioid and non opioid pain killers) might trigger rebound hyperalgesia.

Example 10 : Diuretics (Frusemide , torasemide, triamterene, and others) might cause rebound sodium retention and increased plasma volume leading to elevated blood pressure against which they were used in the first place.

Example 11 : Bronchodilators (short- and long-acting ß-adrenergic agonists, sodium cromoglycate, ipratropium and nedocromil among others) might promote rebound bronchoconstriction with worsening of asthma as paradoxical reaction to discontinuation.

Example 12 : Antiresorptive drugs used for treatment of osteoporosis (denosumab , bisphosphonates, odanacatib and others) might cause paradoxical atypical fractures due to rebound osteoclast activity increase following their discontinuation.

Example 13 : Discontinuation of drugs for treatment of multiple sclerosis (interferon , glucocorticoids, glatiramer acetate, natalizumab, fingolimod, and others) might cause rebound increase of inflammation, with attending exacerbation of clinical symptoms and increase of demyelination lesions.

Example 14 : Immunomodulatory agents (efalizumab and anti-TNFα) indicated for treatment of psoriasis might trigger rebound psoriasis after discontinuation.

Example 15 : Rebound insomnia is insomnia that occurs following discontinuation of sedative substances taken to relieve primary insomnia. Regular use of these substances can cause a person to become dependent on its effects in order to fall asleep. Therefore, when a person has stopped taking the medication and is 'rebounding' from its effects, he or she may experience insomnia as a symptom of withdrawal. Occasionally, this insomnia may be worse than the insomnia the drug was intended to treat.

Dependence liability of Ayurvedic medicines is much less but it must be existing. That is the reason why Ayurvedic textbooks encourage patients not to take some medicines continuously for more than one to two months and to keep gap of 15 days to 1 month before restarting the medicine.
For example , its always better to take Triphala churna in " 2 months on one month off" format to avoid dependence or development of tolerance to its effects.

Since Homeopathy advocates using minimum possible doses of a single well chosen homeopathic medicine and prompt tapering of medicine as soon as substantial response to treatment is noted dependence liability is minimum and incidences of patients becoming physically / mentally dependent on medicine are unheard of.
However , there are examples of initial amelioration of symptoms followed by aggravation of same symptoms during homeopathic treatment. The inference in such cases is that remedy has acted superficially and has palliated the condition. Most likely the remedy was partial similimum. Under such circumstances homeopath has to retake the case in detail with aim of selecting true similimum.

- **<u>Salient features of this rebound effect include :</u>**

1) it induces a body reaction opposed to and of greater intensity compared to the primary action of drugs

2) it takes place after the end of the primary action of the drug or even during therapy if body stops responding to drug (by mechanisms of tachyphylaxis or drug tolerance). The interval between drug discontinuation and appearance of rebound effect is 10 days for salicylates, 14 days for diclofenac , 9 days for rofecoxib , 7 days for statins , 7-14 days for SSRI antidepressants and PPI. In case of deposit drugs (bisphosphonates) this time is longer. The duration of the rebound effect remains for 30 days for rofecoxib , 22 days for SSRI and 30 days for IBP .

3) its magnitude is proportional to the primary action of the drug and

4) it appears in susceptible individuals only (idiosyncrasy).
But since its not possible to predict if it will be seen in a given patient its always advisable to taper the medication slowly , monitor closely and stop cautiously.

Now that we have understood what primary and secondary drug actions are and the phenomenon of rebound effect let us try to answer questions posed above.

Q.1 : *Why Allopathic doctors usually advice patients to take some medicines life long*

A.1 : Because of the rebound phenomenon discussed above

Q.2 : *Why sudden discontinuation of medicines (usually Allopathic ones) leads to reoccurrence of disease in more serious form*

A.2 : Again answer is because of rebound effect.

Q.3 : *What challenges a well intentioned doctor is likely to face when trying to reduce long term medicines of any patient*

A.3 : Suppose a good natured doctor wants to help the patient suffering from multiple health issues and on many different medicines by reducing the number of medicines. His intentions are very noble – reduction in expense on drugs , reduction in long term side effects , reduction in drug interaction and improvement in patient compliance - but is not aware about the complexities of the rebound effect . What will happen? Because of the rebound effect , if above medicines are suddenly stopped and alternative medicines are started patient will experience withdrawal symptoms which may be misattributed to side effects of alternative medicines given. Worsening of clinical situation with development of new symptoms which didn't exist before may occur due to one more mechanism. Suppose a patient is being given multiple Ayurvedic medicines (not being told the names) by Ayurvedic doctor and some of them contain steroids .

Steroids may be lab synthesized or naturally occurring ones with actions same like synthetic steroids. Suppose the new doctor stops these Ayurvedic medicines suddenly . What will happen ? If the patient has been taking these Ayurvedic medicines containing Allopathic steroids or Ayurvedic ingredients with steroid like actions then suppression of HPA (Hypothalamo – Pituitary Axis) might already have occurred. Sudden stoppage would lead to symptoms of adrenal suppression and adrenal crisis (weakness , fatigue , malaise , nausea , vomiting , diarrhoea , myalgia , abdominal pain , fever and anorexia) forcing patient to restart the Ayurvedic medicines. To avoid this complication , the Ayurvedic doctor should be aware of contents and mechanism of action of Ayurvedic medicines and even if he / she does not want to reveal what is being given to the patient , revelation to next doctor must be done.

Q.4 : *Why one needs to always take treatment under proper medical guidance and not self treat , however minor the health issue may be ?*

A.4 : It should be amply clear to any intelligent reader by now that use of medicines even for the simplest of diseases is a highly technical skillfull job and side effects may occur with improper use of medicines for diseases as simple as common cold and cough. Matters are made worse when there is no record of name and dose of medicine (as occurs when patients bypass doctors and take treatment from pharmacist directly or even worse – self medication from internet knowledge) because when problems arise the treating doctor is clueless as to what is producing the difficult to explain symptoms. This problem never arises when treatment is initiated by doctor because then he / she knows what to expect .

Q.5 *Why is there need to integrate the 3 pathies and do intensive research to find out if this integration helps solve the problem of drug dependence ?*

A.5 We have seen many examples above where Allopathic medicines no doubt help a lot in many different diseases but their discontinuation leads to resurgence of same disease in worse form. Since life long intake of medicines is not acceptable to many patients (due to cost factor or side effects) there is need to find solution to the problem. One solution would be to combine Allopathic , Ayurvedic and homeopathic medicines to control the disease symptoms (or cure it). This might minimize cost / side effects and maximum health benefits. Naturally there is need to device new treatment protocols of integrated medicine which can happen only after well designed , well conducted extensive research occurs by tremendous efforts by brilliant doctors of all 3 pathies . These doctors will need to be very highly paid to honour their expertise and provided legal safety in case of any eventuality during research work. Honesty in conducting research and publishing findings as it is should receive topmost importance. Doctors of all 3 pathies should keep aside their preconceived notions and unite together with an open mind for the common aim of devising integrated medicine treatment protocols for various diseases.

So far we have seen 3 points of comparison between the 3 main pathies. Lets now consider the fourth point.

(D) TACHYPHYLAXIS AND DRUG TOLERANCE :

Tachyphylaxis is defined as a rapidly de-creasing response to a drug following its initial administration. On the other hand drug tolerance describes a more gradual loss of response to a drug that occurs over days or weeks.

Mechanisms include :

- reduction in receptors to which the drug binds while producing its effect
- change in the ability of a receptor to affect the downstream signalling molecules
- increased speed of metabolism of the drug and change to inactive metabolites as the liver enzymes become more active.

Psoriasis is one disease where tachyphylaxis and drug tolerance is commonly seen. This frustrates the doctor as well as the patient both of whom feel helpless and perplexed to notice waning off of beneficial effects of medicines which had started to give some benefit. The treating doctor then has no option but to use different weapons in his therapeutic armamentarium. An integrated medical practitioner feels at advantage in such situations because he has many arrows in his therapeutic armamentarium.

<u>Examples of tachyphylaxis and drug tolerance in Allopathic practice :</u>

(1) In ophthalmic practice, the drugs for treating glaucoma and allergic conjunctivitis are the main classes subject to tachyphylaxis.

(2) In psychiatric practice tachyphylaxis and drug tolerance is noted in response to use of anti depressants and anti anxiety medicines.

(3) Another example of drug tolerance is when morphine or alcohol is used for a long time, larger and larger doses must be taken to produce the same effect.

(4) Nicotine may also show tachyphylaxis over the course of a day, although the mechanism of this action is unclear.

(5) Nitroglycerine (or Glyceryl Trinitrate) demonstrates tachyphylaxis when administered transdermally requiring drug-free intervals .

(6) Ranitidine, used for acid reflux treatment, can display rapid tachyphylaxis within six weeks of treatment initiation, limiting its long-term use potential

(7) Drug tolerance may be seen with long term use of ß_2-adrenergic receptor stimulators as bronchodilators. Stimulation results in receptor uncoupling and internalization (desensitization) followed by decrease of the receptor density and downregulation of receptor gene expression . This is seen as lesser and lesser response to bronchodilators with need to use alternative medicines.

<u>Examples of tachyphylaxis and drug tolerance in Ayurvedic practice :</u>

I have not seen the word Tachyphylaxis or drug tolerance being used in English textbooks written on Ayurveda. Tachyphylaxis is not commonly noted in usage of Ayurvedic medicines. Or rather its difficult to note tachyphylaxis when using Ayurvedic medicines because they have slow onset of action and hence its more difficult for patients and doctors to note both onset of action of medicine as well as waning off of their effects.

In Ayurvedic practice something similar to tachyphylaxis is noted in use of laxatives where patients respond lesser and lesser to continuing administration of same dose and require higher and higher dosage of medicines to get same benefit. Keeping this in mind Ayurvedic physicians advice patients to take minimal possible doses of laxatives and encourage patients to intermittently try non drug treatment to enhance bowel movements.

Another example is drug tolerance noted with prolonged use of Ephedra – all parts of this herbal plant are used in Ayurveda as well as ancient Chinese medicine whereas only the top is used in treatment of asthma – Ephedra's most important use.

<u>Examples of tachyphylaxis and drug tolerance in homeopathic practice :</u>

In none of the textbooks of Homeopathy I have read , the word tachyphylaxis or drug tolerance has been mentioned. But - it's a well known fact in Homeopathy - that after few repetitions of correctly selected remedy , patients stop deriving benefit and previously subsided symptoms may recur in mild intensity. The patient is then given a higher potency which once again helps by reducing symptoms and signs of the disease under treatment. I have noted this especially while using Rhus Tox , a remarkable medicine for rheumatic complaints of a particular type and while giving constitutional deep acting therapy for stubborn long standing diseases. In order to speed up the healing process , some homeopaths advocate administration of remedy in ascending potencies (ex. 30 C , 200 C , 1M , 10 M) when diminishing response to successive doses can be anticipated. Needless to say , this therapeutic strategy needs to be closely monitored and fine tuned depending upon patient's response to treatment – and that requires lot of skill and experience.

INTEGRATION OF THE 3 PATHIES :

WHY IS IT ESSENTIAL NOWADAYS TO HAVE ATLEAST BASIC UNDERSTANDING OF ALL 3 PATHIES BY PRACTITIONERS OF ANY PATHY ?

The most important reason why nowadays doctors should have a basic understanding of workings of all 3 pathies is because patients often are simultaneously taking medicines from more than one pathy.

If treating doctor does not have at least a basic knowledge of other pathies SERIOUS blunders can happen in diagnosis and management of the patient. Thus , integrated medical teaching is need of the hour.

I sensed this about 25 years ago and hence started my study of Homeopathy and then of Ayurveda. At that time I was not even aware that there were other allopaths who had studied either Ayurveda or Homeopathy (but I don't know of anyone who has expertise in pathology and working knowledge of all 3 pathies).

The second reason why its always better to have knowledge of all 3 pathies is because it increases therapeutic armamentarium. It's the difference that would be observed when a soldier with limited weapons goes to fight in battlefield versus one who is fully charged with all sorts of weapons. Thus , when patient comes with a disease for which there are no effective treatments in any one pathy , the doctor knowing all 3 pathies can use alternative medical treatments to compensate for this shortcoming.

Example here would be diseases caused by multi drug resistant microbes such as MDR or XDR TB. When no antibiotic is available to which the bacteria are sensitive correctly selected homeopathic medicine will stimulate immunity in such as a way that the bacteria are destroyed and disease cured.

Also , if used very judiciously and carefully , the end result of usage of all 3 pathies might be superior to usage of any one of them. Thus for example , homeopathic medicine will help control excessive sweating and thirst in a patient whose hypertension gets nicely controlled by Allopathic medicines and insomnia gets easily tackled by say Ayurvedic medicines.

There are also a significant number of people today whose diagnosis eludes medical professionals. This usually happens at a very early stage of disease process (in which case Homeopathy has a lot to offer) and at very late stages with numerous complications – where surgery might be the only choice that will work wonders (example renal transplant in chronic renal failure or liver transplant in hepatic failure due to cirrhosis).

The third important reason is need for genuine good quality research into this field of integrated medicine. Currently , articles dealing with studies on efficacy of treatment regimens published in well reputed medical journals pertain to pathy specific treatments. Thus , studies of Allopathic treatment modalities will be found in Allopathic medical journals , Ayurvedic treatment modalities in Ayurvedic medical journals and homeopathic treatment modalities in homeopathic medical journals. THERE ARE HARDLY ANY WELL CONDUCTED STUDIES ON SCIENTIFIC USE OF COMBINATION THERAPIES in patient treatment for various diseases. Hardly any articles are there comparing treatment by say Allopathic medicines for a given disease with treatment by Ayurvedic / homeopathic medicines. Now , even if one were to conduct such studies there would be need of at least one doctor in the research team who has decent working knowledge of all 3 pathies. Such a doctor would play a vital role in trouble shooting problems in designing research studies and help facilitate understanding between doctors of all 3 pathies.

Each of the 3 pathy is so vast that one needs to spend a lifetime before achieving sufficient mastery in ones own field. So intelligent readers can well imagine the extreme hard work and very high intelligence and determination that would be required from a doctor who tries to scientifically study all 3 pathies. It would not be an exaggeration to say that such study would be the most difficult study amongst all studies of everything in this world – medical , engineering , law , finance , arts , political sciences , economics etc etc.

Let me give you few actual clinical examples to highlight how knowledge of all 3 pathies helps in patient management :

Example 1 : I had a patient with primary hypothyroidism (developing after an initial transient phase of hyperthyroidism) who was put on Eltroxine (levothyroxine). Under effect of Eltroxine her TSH levels started declining and came to lie in normal range. For some of her other problems , I treated her using homeopathic medicine which happened to be her constitutional homeopathic medicine. She improved nicely and all her problems were taken care of. After few weeks she started experiencing dyspnoea on accustomed exertion , intermittent episodic palpitations and nervousness. There was no change in her Eltroxine and she was taking her medicine correctly. Because I knew therapeutic benefits of the homeopathic medicine I had given , I correctly diagnosed that homeopathic constitutional medicine must have improved her natural thyroid function so much that previous correct dose of Eltroxine has now become excessive. My suspicion was confirmed by lower than normal TSH and slightly elevated FT3. Reduction in dose of Eltroxine was all that needed to be done and this helped the patient immensely – her dyspnoea , palpitations , nervousness all disappeared. If this history of homeopathic treatment was hidden or if Allopathic doctor would have disregarded homeopathic treatment for want of knowledge , he / she would have got perplexed as to why hyperthyroidism now developed. Thinking of other causes of above symptoms - anemia , asthma , arryhthmias etc - Allopathic doctor would have unnecessarily asked patient to get hemogram , PEFR , 2D Echocardiography , ECG etc to be done.

Example 2 : Patient well controlled by Allopathic medicines for whatever disease , takes poor quality Ayurvedic bhasma (under guidance of Ayurvedic doctor or otherwise) for longer than optimal period of time and slowly develops anemia , tiredness , abdominal pain , tingling numbness , blue line on gums etc. Above could be features of lead toxicity and blood lead level testing would clinch the diagnosis. If treating doctor is aware that lead poisoning or arsenic toxicity is known to occur as a side effect of long term consumption of poorly made Ayurvedic bhasmas then relevant investigations would be asked for and correct diagnosis made.

Example 3 : One patient with intermittent abdominal pain and loose stools without frank diarrhoea was asked by gastroenterologist to get stool examined for occult blood on 3 days. Although a positive occult blood test was expected from gross appearance of the stool , the actual test came repeatedly negative. I knew that large amounts of vitamin C which is a reducing substance can interfere with this test. I was also aware that some Ayurvedic medicines contain large amounts of vitamin C (amla rich preparations). On further digging into the history it became evident that patient was taking large amounts of Vitamin C rich Ayurvedic medicine and did not feel it was important to tell pathologist or gastroenterologist that she was doing so. Thus , entirely because of my knowledge of Ayurveda and Ayurvedic medicines I (an Allopathic doctor and pathologist) was correctly able to pin point the cause behind false negative stool occult blood test in this patient secretly taking Ayurvedic medicines.

Example 4 : Parathyroid hormone (PTH) levels can rise due to Vitamin D deficiency or parenchymal renal disease with renal failure (Secondary hyperparathyroidism) or rarely due to parathyroid pathology (adenomas , carcinomas , hyperplasias) – a condition referred to as primary hyperparathyroidism. PTH is catabolized to some metabolic intermediates and commonly available hormone analyzers not only measure the entire PTH hormone but also these metabolic intermediates. Further , since these metabolic intermediates accumulate in blood in chronic renal failure , PTH levels are reported disproportionately high. I had a patient with both severe vitamin D deficiency and renal failure. His PTH was very high and because of some complex lab related technical issues hypercalcemia was wrongly reported in him. Primary hyperparathyroidism is responsible for 99.9% of cases having this combination of very high PTH with hypercalcemia. Sestamibi scans revealed normal parathyroid glands – which ruled out primary hyperparathyroidism. Upon advise by some friend , he started homeopathic treatment and within just a few days his PTH reduced drastically. It would be wrong to conclude that homeopathic treatment helped in primary hyperparathyroidism because sestamibi scans failed to reveal parathyroid pathology. But here it is important to note in history that vitamin D supplements were given to tackle its deficiency. Further , on enquiry it was noted that homeopathic treatment helped drastically improve the renal function. Thus the beneficial effect noted in form of reduction of PTH levels could be attributed to rectification of vitamin D deficiency (credit to Allopathy) and improvement in renal function (credit to Homeopathy). This example also highlights the fact that sound knowledge of technical complexities of pathology testing and therapeutics can totally change interpretation of what is observed in clinical practice.

As a summary , patients nowadays use medicines for more than one pathy and hence a doctor trained in integrated medicine would always have an edge over one who has absolutely no idea of workings of other 2 pathies besides his own pathy. There is urgent need for genuine high quality research into practical aspects of polypathy in day to day clinical practice.

"Alternative Health Care" is becoming a misnomer. There is so much inclination of patients nowadays to try out non Allopathic treatment modalities primarily or at least to "complement" current Allopathic treatment with Ayurveda or Homeopathy that they along with other alternative treatment modalities" should rather be called "Complementary Medicine".

The integration of complementary and conventional therapies would not necessarily mean that they would be used at the same time on a patient. Rather , there will be times only modern medicine will be indicated and other times when only Ayurveda / Homeopathy will be indicated and still other times when all 3 would be indicated together. The decisions on when to use each would naturally be taken by doctors having knowledge of potentials of all 3 pathies and as all are aware there are but handful of such doctors at present time.

PRACTICE OF INTEGRATED MEDICINE IN FUTURE WOULD POSE NEW CHALLENGES :
Currently , there is no undergraduate or post graduate course in integrated medicine anywhere in the world – atleast I am not aware of any country having such a course. Even if a new course of integrated medicine was to be started there would be many challenges in the whole process.

Challenge 1 : First and foremost would be to form committees of doctors of each of the 3 pathies to set forth framework and guidelines for designing a course of integrated medicine. There would be need to come out with a separate degree – for example BIMS (Bachelor of Integrated Medicine and Surgery). Its likely that expert academicians may recommend to the government that rather than keeping this as a bachelors course , it should be kept as a masters degree course after bachelors degree in any of the 3 pathies (MBBS , BAMS and BHMS). Doctors passing such a specially designed course may be awarded MIM degree
(Masters in Integrated Medicine).

Challenge 2 : Further challenge would be establishment of medical colleges teaching integrated medicine and hospitals affiliated to them having staff skilled in use of integrated medicine. The patients who come to these hospitals would know before hand that they are likely to receive treatment from one or more of these pathies.
Since post graduate doctors are expected to write and present a thesis on any topic , creation of a masters course would definitely encourage fundamental research in integrated medicine. For this research to be of good caliber , government or some third party needs to fund such a research : resident doctors salary , guide's salary , expenses on research work etc

Challenge 3 : Next challenge would be establishment of regulatory bodies looking after registration of doctors trained in integrated medicine . There would be need to design CME programs specific to integrated medicine.

Challenge 4 : Law may need to be amended to give legal protection to doctors of integrated medicine. This would be of paramount importance at least during initial few decades when research in designing of integrated medicine treatment protocols would be in its infancy. Otherwise out of fear of law suits and punishment no doctor would be willing to get enrolled in degree courses of integrated medicine and the entire idea will flop.

BONUS SECTION

Articles on pathology lab testing and doctor patient interaction and some other related topics for non medicos primarily.

ARTICLE 1: THROUGH THE SKY GAZERS EYES

Dear Patron

First of all , I ….Dr. Amol Javdekar would like to sincerely thank you for the trust you have shown in me as pathologist and for appreciating services provided to you.

To strengthen this bond of relationship between you and me , good communication is essential and hence I write these articles for you with the purpose of **clearing certain misconceptions about pathology lab testing , financial aspects of medical services , challenges facing medical fraternity , doctor patient relationship etc . etc. etc.**

Even before I go ahead , I want to make it very clear that **<u>pathology and the entire field of medicine is horribly , painfully complex</u>** and it would be next to impossible to educate non medicos about the intricacies and finer nuances of diagnosis and treatment of any disease in a span of few words. However , even if the reader gets an overview of this challenging field of medicine and understand why certain things need to be done the way they are done , one can consider these articles to have served their purpose.

This is somewhat like staring at a star studded sky. From a distance all stars look the same. But look at them through a telescope ….. and ….. the finer details of the stars and differences between them will become apparent. **<u>Thus things remain the same , but perceptions about them change when we look at them more closely</u>**. What is true for the star studded sky , is equally true for the challenges studded field of medicine. Look at these articles as a telescope (or as a microscope) which will take you closer to reality pertaining to the field of medicine , and , in particular , pathology lab testing.

The most common questions that come to minds of patients undergoing a series of diagnostic tests are :

Q.1 : Are all these tests really required ?

Q.2 : Where should I get these tests done from ?

Q.3 : How much (or why so much) is the cost of testing ?

Q.4 : Why are there differences in values of tests between path labs ?

Q.5 : Why am I being asked to repeat a particular test ?

and so on and so forth.

As I answer each of these questions , I will try to keep the language as simple as possible. To understand certain issues pertaining to lab testing , technical information is required and there are **limitations to how technical this discussion can be.**

ARTICLE 2: BASICS OF PATHOLOGY LAB TESTING : PART 1

Hello Friends

We are just beginning on our journey and trying to understand answers to following questions……

> **WHY TO DO PATHOLOGY LAB TESTING IN THE FIRST PLACE ?**

The **most common question** that comes to the minds of even educated people is : I am not experiencing any symptoms , then **why should I un necessarily get tested : spend the time , money and energy on the same ?** To anyone who has this question in his or her mind I would like to ask few questions which provide insight into this issue :

Q.1 : Haven't you ever heard of comments like : Mr So and so was so hale and hearty and doing all his routine work and all of a sudden he had a heart attack and expired. He was just , say 40 + ……. such a young age to die ?

Q.2 : Haven't you heard comments from patients that they were experiencing seemingly minor complaints like repeated early morning headache , ignored that assuming that to be tension headache and were shocked when MRI done revealed an advanced brain tumour ?

Q.3 : Haven't you heard of people saying that they are non alcoholic , non smokers , don't have any serious complaints apart from recurrent nausea , gas trouble and were surprised to find path lab report stating deranged liver function tests ?

To be honest , we all have heard of many such real life incidences , **but love to believe that such things happen only to others , not to us. We would rather enjoy bliss in ignorance than come face to face with an underlying medical condition** , however trivial it may be.

Such incidences occur because **in the early stage of development , majority of diseases produce either no symptoms or produce minor symptoms** which patients prefer to ignore rather than follow up. That's one reason behind getting your routine annual health checkup.

The other reason is …….. **importance of baseline values of any test i.e patients own result of a test when he apparently has absolutely no reason for an abnormal value for that test**. Let me explain this further in the form of an example. Let us say , that normal hemoglobin range for adult Indian females is 12 – 16 gm%. Suppose one particular female's baseline normal hemoglobin is 16 gm% but is not known to her because she never got it tested. She develops something known as a hemolytic process in which because of some disease her RBCs start getting broken down. Due to this her hemoglobin starts falling , becomes 15 then 14 , then 13 gm% and by chance she presents to the pathologist at a stage when her hemoglobin is 13 gm%. In a very busy pathology lab , where pathologist has no access to patient's complaints , there are less chances that the pathologist will think of a hemolytic process with a Hb of 13 gm%. On the other hand , if the baseline normal of 16 gm% is known and compared to the current 13 gm% , the pathologist will note a significant drop of 3 gm% of hemoglobin and view peripheral smear carefully , do certain other tests and correctly pick up this disease at an early stage.

What applies to hemoglobin applies equally to almost all other tests. Hence , next time when you get your pathology lab testing from a good lab and get normal results , don't feel it has been a waste of your time and money. **Be happy that you have got good results and have got to know your own baseline values.** There are certain other complexities in this issues ….. but I will not bore you with discussion of those.

➤ **FREQUENCY OF PATHOLOGY LAB TESTING :**

Patients go to pathology lab either for routine **yearly health checkup** or if they have been asked to get some tests done by their treating doctor.

As far as yearly health checkup is concerned , between the **ages 40 – 60 yrs** it is always advisable to get certain basic tests done **once every year**. **Post 60 yrs** , relevant clinical examination and diagnostic testing need to be done **twice a year**. This would definitely **help early detection of a subclinical disease process.**

The actual tests that need to be done can be advised by the clinician or even by the pathologist , who also is first a clinician and then a pathologist by training. **A proper history and clinical examination will guide the doctor which tests to advice** and hence remember , friends , **don't seek free medical advice on phone , but rather seek a proper consultation from your trusted doctor for the same. Let the doctor know before hand that you are visiting him for a paid consultation.**

➤ **WHY AM I BEING ASKED TO REPEAT A PATH LAB TEST :**

Majority of the times , your treating doctor or the pathologist does not ask you to repeat the path tests already done. The **scientifically correct reasons** why doctors may be justified in asking for a repeat testing are as follows :

1. **A borderline result :** repetition is required to look for trends in values which will help making a correct diagnosis…. Otherwise a normal person with a result lying outside **" population normal range "** would be wrongly diagnosed as being diseased

2. **An unexpected result not matching with clinical picture :** obviously both clinicians and pathologist wonder if any error has occurred in reporting and hence just to be sure that there was no error in testing a repeat testing is asked for
3. **During follow up to evaluate response to treatment given :** Suppose you have an abnormally high cholesterol level and physician gives you a medicine to reduce that level back to normal range…. Under such circumstances , obviously a repeat testing is asked for **to assess response to treatment and need to stop treatment.**

> **TIPS TO GET THE MOST OUT OF PATH LAB TESTING :**

Tip 1: Carry all your previous reports done in any diagnostic center and show to the technician / pathologist. If any tests have been repeated , make a table showing changes in values of that analyte over period of time.

Tip 2 : Even if lab staff do not ask you on their own , do **tell about your present symptoms and any treatment** (including Ayurvedic , homeopathic , home remedies etc) and see to it that this information is mentioned on test requisition form. In case of an abnormal , unexpected value , this will save valuable efforts for the lab staff in trying to contact you for the desired information. Note that medicines that you may be taking can directly influence accuracy and reliability of lab reports. **How well information provided by you is correlated with the lab and other results depends upon knowledge and skill of the pathologist.**

Tip 3 : Please get path lab test done as soon as the clinician asks you to do so. It's a common tendency to postpone path lab testing. Remember , what the clinician is trying to do is to co relate the symptoms you have told him with path lab results. **Values of some analytes keep on changing and hence if you show test report done after a few days it may not co relate with clinical suspicion physician had when he examined you and it will be sheer waste of your money.** Also note that since one cannot go back in time , the diagnostic opportunity lost is lost forever.

Tip 4 : Never ever…. I repeat …. never ever get pathology lab testing done from technician run labs or from any lab where pathologist just signs reports without actually supervising the processing of samples. I will go into details of this issue in a subsequent article.

ARTICLE 3: BASICS OF PATHOLOGY LAB TESTING : PART 2

Hello Friends

Let us continue our discussion about some basic aspects of path lab testing with this article.

> **WHY DO RESULTS VARY BETWEEN TWO DIFFERENT LABS ?**

A **common question** asked by patients who keep on shifting between labs to do their tests is : **I got the same analyte tested from two different labs and the actual values have come out to be different. Why so ?**

If I am asked this question the first thing that I do is to ensure that apples are compared with apples and not oranges. This I do by taking a careful look at :

- **what analyte is the patient complaining about :** most common mistakes are comparing results of :

- free T3/ free T4 with results of Total T3 / Total T4
- GHB with HbA1c

- **is there difference in the method used to evaluate the analytes :** most common mistakes are comparing :

- Alkaline phosphatase done by one method with that done by another method
- LDL estimated by formula versus direct LDL estimation

- **is there difference in the factors related to sample collection :** most common mistakes are comparing :

- FSH , LH , Prolactin done during end of m.c with that done on 3rd day of m.c
- HBsAg positivity noted early after infection with its negativity after development of anti HBsAg antibodies (something which is to be expected)
- Widal negativity in first few days of fever with its positivity say during second week of fever

Next thing to do is see if the inferences given by two reports are different : for example , whether results of one lab suggest hypothyroidism and that from other lab where testing was done just the next day is suggesting hyperthyroidism. If there is agreement in the inferences , then I tell patients not to go into the details of minor differences in values. **However , if the inferences are opposite or same but with markedly differing values then there is a high chance that one of the result in wrong. Which one is wrong depends upon individual case.**

Have you heard about random variability ? You would be surprised to know that if you were to run a sample on one machine in one particular lab and after a short delay run the same sample on the same machine in the same lab , a minor difference in values is to be expected. In technical terms we refer to this as **random variability which is there in all labs and applies to almost all analytes.**

Differences in test results between two labs can occur because of following reasons :

[A] FACTORS OPERATING EVEN BEFORE SAMPLE IS TAKEN :

• **Diurnal (daily) variation :** For example , most hormones , CBC values etc show diurnal variation i.e even normally these values fluctuate during the day. Thus , for example , suppose an absolutely normal person gets his hemogram and serum cortisol done from one lab early in the morning , disapproves of the report and gets the same tests done say in the evening from another lab , a difference in results is to be expected for no fault of either of the labs.

- **Fasting / non fasting status**
- **Position of patient** (sleeping / standing for long time etc)
- **Day of menstrual cycle in females**
- **Response to treatment given** (Allopathic, Ayurvedic, homeopathic,home remedies)
- **Altitude of the place from sea level**
- **Variable influences of combination of more than one disease present**

[B] FACTORS OPERATING AT THE TIME SAMPLE IS TAKEN :

These include :

- Patient **correctly identified or not** and whether sample enters appropriate container
- How **tightly or how long tourniquet** has been applied
- Prior warming of limb or not
- Whether patient was able to correctly follow instructions given by lab staff : this especially applies to urine sample (where patient may not submit mid stream sample) , sputum (where patient may submit saliva or saliva mixed sputum) , semen (where patient may find it difficult to give sample within lab premises)
- Blood sample collected in single prick / multiple pricks and whether this led to hemolysis or not

[C] FACTORS OPERATING WHILE SAMPLE IS BEING PROCESSED :

These include :

- Whether sample is correctly fed into machine
- Whether **proper quality control** has been done before running sample
- **Jaundiced , hemolyzed , turbid** samples likely to give incorrect results
- Variation in electric power supply while machine is operating

- Diligence of pathologist or technician in following S.O.Ps

[D] FACTORS OPERATING AFTER SAMPLE ANAYSIS IS OVER :
These include :
- By chance **2 patients having same name** so that reports of one typed for other
- <u>**Typing errors by the typist**</u>
- <u>**Interpretation errors by patient , clinician , pathologist**</u>
- Failure to look at methodology , timing of sample in relation to disease process , **failure to look at units** etc.

Friends , tell me honestly … do you think all these factors would get addressed in any lab where pathologist is either absent (technician run lab) or present part time ?
It must be clear by now that answering your seemingly simple query requires so much efforts from lab side. **So , please value the pathologists efforts / expertise by offering due fees for seeking his / her consultation and do not demand this opinion for free. Make this clear right at the beginning of your conversation with the pathologist.**
In fact , if the pathologist anticipates that you are not going to pay , he may not give sufficient time to your query and just answer something of no use out of inability to say no.

➤ **HOW TO SELECT A GOOD PATHOLOGY LAB ?**
Most patients would actually like to zero in on one good pathology lab and do all investigations in that lab for the rest of their lives. Actually this is a correct practice and since we are talking about a **long term association** , I will provide you with what to and what not to consider while selecting a pathology lab.

What to consider while selecting a pathology lab to trust your health with ?
1. Most important criteria is it should be a pathologist run lab with a full time (atleast 8 hrs) pathologist under whose supervision all lab work is done. Technicians are meant to assist pathologist in lab work and Indian law does not permit technicians to sign pathology reports. To circumvent this legal hurdle and make money , most technicians who own labs have part time pathologist who does not see how the tests are done and just signs reports without verifying their reliability. Even worse , these technicians force pathologists to give pre-signed letterheads on which reports are printed without pathologist knowledge.
Now you will ask : how to know whether the lab from which I have been getting myself checked has a full time pathologist or not.

Since you are paying for the services provided by your lab you have every right to verify who is the owner of the lab. Just take out one day. Go to the lab multiple times during the day and skillfully , without letting the lab staff come to know , see if pathologist is there inside the lab and whether lab testing is being done under his/her supervision. You would be shocked to know that some pathologists give presigned reports or inadequately tested reports to 50+ labs. Just think logically , can any pathologist work at more than 2 – 3 labs and do justice to such a technically challenging work ?

2. **Natural tendency is to select a path lab closest to your home or office.** For practical reasons also its better to do so. But , if such a lab does not meet the above criteria , you must change the lab.

3. **If the lab has NABL accreditation / ISO certification all the more better.** Although its the only objective way of assessing lab quality , give more importance to your own experience with the lab , how satisfied you are with the services provided , rather than any such logo on lab reports.

4. **Pathologist with sound clinical knowledge :** There are very few pathologists who also do general practice i.e they actually ask history to the patient , clinically examine the patient and then advice pathology / radiology tests to confirm or refute the tentative diagnosis. I personally feel that such is the best possible situation because such a doctor constantly improves his own clinical and pathology knowledge and gives better , more reliable reports.

ARTICLE 4 : IMPROVING DOCTOR - PATIENT RELATIONSHIP

Hello Friends

In today's article I am going to discuss with you a practically important aspect of pathology work and that is : **Improvement of Doctor – Patient relationship.**

An **ideal relationship** between path lab and patient should be one of **total trust , satisfaction and gratitude from both sides.**

But is this the picture we see nowadays ? We see path labs giving fake reports , we see patients hiding information from path labs , we see path labs behaving in a mechanical fashion with patients and we see patients duping pathology lab of their well deserved fees. What has given rise to such an unwanted situation ? Frankly , both patients and path lab staff are to be blamed for this.

There are certain duties which patients and path lab staff have towards each other and some rights which they should enjoy. Let us see what these are

[A] DUTIES OF PATIENTS TOWARDS PATHOLOGY LAB :

1. Once an appointment is taken please stick to it.

Often it so happens that patients take an appointment with the path lab or clinician , speak to the pathologist / clinician , inform lab about tests to be done and then fail to turn up as promised and when asked give some flimsy reason.

This is not fair. **You , as a patient , must value the path lab / clinician's time.** At times , even without your knowing the path lab or pathologist may be making some personal sacrifices to ensure that you get the best of services and then when you don't turn up all these sacrifices go waste.

In your own profession would you like your clients not abiding by the given appointment ? Definitely not …. right ? Then please don't miss a path lab appointment for any flimsy , false reason.

2. Be sincere about your own health and follow the doctors advice

In my experience I have encountered **3 types of patients : first category of those who are excessively obsessed with their health , second category** where the patients are **very casual and not bothered** about their own health and the **third (the ideal one) where patients show optimum concern about their health**. It is the third category of patients who benefit maximum from healthcare industry.

At times, a caring , dedicated pathologist spends so much time in explaining the tests and need to do them and patients say yes to everything on his / her face and then do just as they please.

Some patients don't even bother to collect the path lab report. I wonder , why they spend money to do investigations in the first place if they are not bothered to collect reports .

If your treating physician gives you a set of advice follow it exactly …. don't forget his advice and modify the treatment as per your convenience. **If you don't follow doctors advice , you have no right to blame him / her for not getting desired results.**

3. Offer fees for consultation , investigations and treatment.

Make it clear to the clinician / pathologist / radiologist , right at the beginning of your interactions with him / her that you are **not expecting free services and are willing to pay for consultation in addition to testing and treatment** (medicines / equipments etc). Some patients willingly dupe pathology lab of test charges / pathologists consultation fees.

4. Please ensure regular follow untill you recover completely

95% of the times patients don't bother to give feedback (honest feedback … both positive and negative as the case may be) to the doctor regarding efficacy of treatment / correctness of lab reports. Please note , dear patients , that such a **feedback received from each and every patient to whom advice is given by any doctor enriches his / her experience and makes him / her a better doctor.** Any when all doctors improve because of timely patient feedback who is going to benefit the most – the patients obviously … right ?

Unlike mathematics , medicine is not a 100% science. In maths 2+ 2 is always 4 , in medicine it can be 3 or 5. Further , every human being is different than any other….unlike say cars of one make …. 1000th car of a particular model manufactured by the assembly line technique is exactly the same as 1st ………. not so with human beings….. each of the quadrillions of humans manufactured by GOD is different and the human body is thousand times more complex than design of an automobile……….., the possibilities of causes of malfunctioning of cars are limited but too many as far as human body is concerned. And hence , your feedback is very valuable to him / her to understand your body which is unique to you and not shared by anyone else.

 And there are so many other issues apart from the human body which influence disease process and response to treatment. Needless to say , doctors face a lakh times more challenging situations in their day to day work as compared to other professionals.

[B] DUTIES OF DOCTORS TOWARDS PATIENTS :

1. Give adequate time to properly examine each and every patient

Nowadays , patients often complain that doctors don't give them sufficient time , just ask a few hurried questions and do a cursory examination and then give them a long list of investigations or scribble down some medicines without explaining how to take them.. .. obviously this is not true for many doctors … but , sadly , for many other doctors these patient complaints hold true.

It is duty of the treating doctor , to first take a proper history , do a thorough clinical examination and then formulate some differential diagnosis and then order pathology / radiological investigations to confirm / rule out these differential diagnosis.

And if this takes a lot of time , it is perfectly fair for the doctor to demand proportionate fees from the patient. In fact , the best thing to do is to keep consultation charges as Rs. XYZ per 15 minutes , per 5 minutes or so.

2. A gentle and human approach is needed

As any other Indian citizen , the doctor may be having his / her own problems and frustrations in life . But these should not influence behavior towards any patient , i.e doctor should not vent his frustrations on patients.

It is the duty of the doctor to be kind , compassionate and human in dealing with all patients. Be sensitive to the pain / discomfort experienced by patient while he is being examined / investigated. Give your total undivided attention to the patient.

3. Explain test results clearly :

In case a patient wants to understand pathology / radiology report the diagnostician should explain the same without making any fuss. However , if this is going to take a lot of time and recurring advice is necessary then the patient should volunteer to pay some nominal fees to diagnostician as consultation charges.

4. Explain treatment strategy clearly :

It's the duty of treating doctor to explain treatment strategy is simple , clear language and ensure that patient has followed what he / she wants to say. Prescriptions should be written in easily readable hand writing and clear instructions should be given regarding follow up. There should be no compulsion on the patient to get tests done from any particular lab (only condition should be that it should be a pathologist run lab) or for branded medicines (only condition should be that generic medicines if taken should be of good quality as per doctors previous experience with them).

5. Give a tentative idea of total expenses likely :
Its difficult for the doctor to give idea of total expenses till he has got a crystal clear idea of what the patient is suffering from and what treatment modalities are available to treat that condition. But once that information is available , the treating doctor should try his / her level best to give a tentative estimate of total expenses likely to be incurred as accurately as possible.
With both patient and doctors following their duties and giving respect to each other , the goodness and freshness of this doctor patient relationship can once again be revived.

ARTICLE 5 : UNDERSTANDING FINANCIAL ASPECTS OF MEDICAL PRACTICE

Hello Friends

Now , lets discuss an exceedingly important aspect of medical practice and that is … the financial aspect.

> **WHAT ARE THE EXPENSES THAT THE DOCTORS FACE IN THEIR PRACTICE ?**

One very important thing that patients must remember whenever they pay fees in hospital / lab is that all the money they pay don't go to the doctors who treat / care for them .
There are so many expenses to be taken care of :

1. electricity bills

2. telephone bills

3. municipal taxes , income tax and other taxes

4. security

5. salaries of technicians / nurses / ward boys / office staff / security staff / doctors / administrators etc etc

6. Recurring expenses on stationary and other consumables

7. If loan is taken then loan E.M.I

8. Cuts or reference charges which go back to referring clinician if business is generated from cut practice. This is sad but true state of affairs.

9. Professional indemnity insurance premium

10.   Cost of staying up to date in knowledge. This is quite unique to medical profession because constant improvements are taking place in treatment modalities. Doctors need to complete some clock hours of CME programs and earn credit points (all of which need to be paid from own pocket) in order to remain registered with state medical councils.

Don't ever forget that profit has to be made over and above these expenses for the commercial entity to survive. Other wise your most trusted healthcare center and your favourite doctor would soon have to shut down business.

➤ **DO DIFFERENCES IN EXPENSES ACCOUNT FOR DIFFERENCES IN DOCTORS FEES ?**

Its really unfortunate that people go "doctor shopping" the way they go vegetable shopping. Comparing prices of pathology lab tests between two labs is not the same as comparing prices of vegetables between two vegetable vendors.

Due consideration has to be given to following points :

- **Expenses incurred by doctor in getting his / her medical education :**

I will put forth in front of you 4 categories under which student doctors bear expenses of medical education and then will ask you a question. These four categories are :

1. A reserved category candidate whose entire medical education (including book expenses and hostel fees) is almost free being taken care of government using honest tax payers money

2. A non reserved category candidate who has spent thousands of rupees for fees and incidental expenses (book s, hostel etc) in government college

3. A candidate who has spent a few lakhs for getting education in private medical college through government seat quota

4. A candidate who has paid a hefty donation to owners of medical colleges for seeking medical education through management quota in medical colleges and whose expense reach almost half a crore or even one crore rupees.

Assuming all the 4 candidates are same in merit , for the sake of discussion , how do you expect each of the 4 doctors to charge same fees for the same service provided ?

In fact , is it fair , on part of the patient to do so ?

- **Seniority and experience of the doctor**

In government setup , government employees get dearness allowance and seniority benefits whether their workload increases proportionate to increase in salary or not.

On the other hand , private practice doctors (clinician or diagnostician) having vastly different experience (novice to say 30 + years experience) are expected to charge same fees. Not fair… isn't it ?

- **Area in which the doctor practices**

The cost of purchasing a clinic , taking it on rent , expenses on items of daily living differ vastly amongst rural areas and city area and between different localities within the same city. These need to be factored in while deciding cost of various services provided by healthcare setup.

These are just a few major expenses that doctors and managers of healthcare setups incur to remain operational. Profit has to be made over and above these expenses to survive. There is a vast difference in operational costs for a charitable venture and a for profit hospital and in the absence of this knowledge opinions are formed by media and general public alike. Having said that , exploitation of patients by unnecessary testing and therapeutic procedures also takes place. So … in short .. all is not well with healthcare industry and one really needs to make judgements on case to case basis.

ARTICLE 6 : FOR YOUR OWN SAKE DON'T COMMIT THESE MISTAKES

Hello Friends

In this article , I will be discussing certain mistakes committed by patients while trying to get better from disease . Steer clear of these self detrimental practices.

MISTAKE 1 : RELYING ON INTERNET AND SOCIAL MEDIA FOR MEDICAL KNOWLEDGE

Although internet has revolutionized accessibility to a universe of information , lack of control of this information and lack of regulation by experts makes the information undependable and risky to health.

The situation is somewhat similar to mainstream media (newspapers) and social media. There are more chances that information printed in newspapers would be reliable and authentic as compared to information posted on social media (whatts app , facebook , twitter etc) because the former is more regulated and answerable to law.

Most medical information on internet and social media is either completely or partially false. Its written by anyone who has something to gain : financially or otherwise from posting that information. In order to catch hold of your attention , medical facts are distorted , glorified and put forth in a catchy attractive manner – with no efforts taken to ensure truthfulness of the statements made. For example : suppose there are 5 studies done worldwide 3 of which show a small benefit of consuming dark chocolate by heart disease patients and 2 showing absolutely no such correlation.

How should this information be truthfully made public ?

Benefit of eating dark chocolate by heart patients is small and that too controversial.

How is this information actually made public to general public ?

Go and grab that enticing piece of dark chocolate – new study shows that it really benefits heart disease patients.

See the difference ?

In the above example , manufacturers of dark chocolate would stand to benefit by spread of such (wrong) information in public as their sales will increase.

You will say – that even doctors have access to such information and can be fooled by such wrong information. True to some extent …. but there are 2 differences.

1. Good , knowledgeable doctors can evaluate both sides of the coin by accessing these studies in medical journals and read expert critical analysis of all studies (meta- analysis)

2. With patients permission , actually employ any of these treatments to verify their

truthfulness. As the experience of doctor builds up , he / she will be in far better position to comment on authenticity of such tall claims.

Patients don't just read information on internet but indulge in following unhealthy practices
1. Take a sort of examination of doctor by asking questions about recently read information and challenge doctors who tell anything patient does not want to hear
2. Self medicate , hide information from doctors / nurses and risk overdosing / side effects of wrong medication
3. Begin imagining side effects (when actually nothing is happening) by reading them on internet.

The health hazards from above practices are obvious but what is not so obvious is the bitterness and suspicion it brings in the doctor – patient relationship which should be based on mutual trust and respect.

And hence I urge you , dear patients , **<u>NOT TO TAKE ANY INFORMATION ON INTERNET OR SOCIAL MEDIA AT FACE VALUE AND NEVER TO TAKE HEALTH RELATED DECISIONS FROM SUCH INACCURATE KNOWLEDGE.</u>**

MISTAKE - 2 : SELF MEDICATE OR TAKE OTC MEDICINES WITHOUT CONSULTING THE DOCTOR

Unlike in US / Europe there is easy access to doctors in India. Also healthcare practices are far more flexible and much much cheaper than abroad. In spite of these facts , some patients (especially the under educated and those from lower socio – economic strata) , bypass the doctors when they fall sick and tend to take medicines directly from the pharmacy. The pharmacist (busy with other customers and in a situation which is not at all ideal for detailed case taking) just asks one or two questions and gives whatever medicine comes to his mind. No history is taken about drug allergies , no attempt is made to make a proper diagnosis , proper instructions of taking medicines are not given , no attempt is made to safeguard against possible interactions with other medicines the patient may be taking and absolutely no record is kept of treatment given.

What all can go wrong due to this unhealthy practice?
1. Since there are no records of history taken or clinical examination findings , that opportunity to document this very important information is lost forever.
   Further since no diagnosis is made and if symptoms don't subside - no one will know what was the diagnosis at the precise moment when OTC medicines were taken ---

because the medicines would have already altered patient's health status by the
time he / she now presents to a properly qualified doctor.

2. Giving a medicine to which patient is allergic even by chance can be fatal. There have been
incidences of deaths due to taking medicine to which patient is allergic as a over the
counter medicine from pharmacist.

3. Patient takes medicine directly from pharmacist for just 1 or 2 days. There is no record
of what medicine was given. Patient does not feel well and now goes to a well qualified
doctor. Tells doctor that some medicine was given by pharmacist. Which one ? Not known.
Now the doctor is in fix.
Since the medicine has not worked , there is no point in giving the same medicine ?
But wait … which medicine was given ?
No idea … as no record was kept. Doctor now gives some medicine after examining
the patient. 3 things can happen :
(1) patient feels better and gets cured
(2) drug interaction occurs between the doctors medicine and unknown pharmacist
    medicine leading to new symptoms (difficult to decide whether due to drug
    interaction or part of disease process) or
(3) overdose occurs because of chance administration of same medicine. For example
    patient takes 3 capsules of 60,000 IU of vitamin D and doctor administers 6 lakh
    IU of architol injection not knowing oral Vit - D has been given ….. leading to
    vitamin D toxicity.

4. Medicine given by pharmacist can interfere with results of pathology tests. This can
of course happen with medicine given by doctor… but in that case pathologist can
speak with treating doctor and enquire about administration of any medicine known
to interfere with path lab test results.

5. Patient shows empty strip of medicine to different pharmacies and keeps on taking
medicine just because he feels better from it. With the help of an example lets see
how this can endanger patient's health. If this medicine happens to be a steroid ,
patient will develop overdosage side effects because of long term intake and because
of suppression of brain level controls can land into ICU if care is not taken to taper
down the medicine before stopping.

I have seen at least 2 patients who have landed themselves into almost incurable medicine induced diseases by long term intake of medicines taken over the counter - directly from pharmacist. So, to conclude on this, dear patient, as far as possible do not self treat by taking medicines directly from pharmacist.

MISTAKE- 3 : EXPECT INSTANT RESULTS FOR ALL DISEASES AND KEEP ON CHANGING DOCTORS IN AN IMPATIENT MANNER

Today we are all living in an "instant" era. We are so much accustomed to instant services and results in non medical issues that we tend to expect the same from medical treatment when we fall ill.

Its ok to expect results in a few days for acute conditions like seasonal cold, cough, fever etc. But long standing, slowly developing chronic health issues like osteoarthritis, rheumatoid arthritis, varicose veins, skin problems etc need to be given time to heal and "patient" has to be "patient" and not expect instant results.

If your doctor has taken a proper history, examined you thoroughly, explained treatment protocol to you nicely and you trust his intentions … please DO NOT CHANGE your doctor just because you don't get well in just a few days. **Always follow up with same doctor and give exact feedback**. At time what happens is both diagnosis and treatment are actually correct, but **because of genetic considerations that medicine does not suit the patient well.** For example, let us say one particular medicine on oral intake gets absorbed into blood stream and is converted into active medicine by liver in body of 99% of all people. You may be the unfortunate 1% whose liver can not convert that correctly selected medicine into an active medicine. Naturally you will not benefit from that medicine. But obviously this is not fault of the treating doctor.

Lets take another example of …. say …. medicines to help reduce cravings for alcohol. Different people get benefitted from different anti craving medicines and no doctor can predict in advance which medicine will benefit. Trial and error needs to be done under such circumstances. **Please trust your doctor and give him the opportunity to change medicine and find out what works best for you.**

Another reason is – especially true for homeopathic treatment – if constitutional holistic treatment is being given for diseases that are as chronic as a few decades – it can take months of continuous treatment to get well totally. Its' the treating doctor's duty to give a realistic idea of this to the patient right at start of treatment so that the patient prepares himself / herself mentally for a long term treatment.

Here , I would like to emphasize another facet of this issue. Medicine is an ever changing branch and years after doctors pass out of medical colleges new medicines and treatments keep on being invented. If such treatments are evaluated on sufficiently large number of patients with promising results , they get mentioned in newer editions of medicine textbooks. So , if the doctor has tried to give you a cheaper medicine about which he has in depth knowledge and if it fails to work as expected , you should give your doctor another chance to use a newer (but costlier) treatment modality. As far as possible , if you trust your doctor and he is genuinely interested in your well being don't change him un necessarily.

MISTAKE - 4 FROM PATIENTS : HIDING OF INFORMATION
There is a saying : Don't hide anything from the doctor and lawyer. And that's really true. Hiding of any information from your doctor can be detrimental to you as far as your health is concerned.
At times patient may not give accurate information to doctor for few reasons :
1. Not understood what doctor is asking or misunderstanding doctors question and not realizing question has been misunderstood.
2. Purposeful hiding of information due to shame or guilt or other ulterior motive.
3. Memory problems : especially true in elderly individuals and on those who are intellectually challenged.
How can this be detrimental to patient's health and wellbeing ?
1. By hiding information , an important feature essential for diagnosis may be lost for consideration
2. If information about medicines (Allopathic , Ayurvedic , home remedies , dietary supplements) is not told to doctor there are chances of drug interactions developing when doctor prescribes medicines in absence of this vital knowledge
To make patient feel at ease and to help maintain confidentiality about health related information it may be necessary to examine patient one to one (without presence of relatives or friends).

These are just few of the important oft repeated mistakes patients commit – knowingly or unknowingly and land themselves into trouble. For your own good – steer clear from them.

With that dear readers we come to end of this book.
Requesting your honest feedback via mobile call , whatts app or email.